Intensive Care Infections

A PRACTICAL GUIDE TO DIAGNOSIS AND MANAGEMENT IN ADULT PATIENTS

Hilary Humphreys MD FRCPI FRCPath
Consultant and Professor of Microbiology
Royal College of Surgeons in Ireland and Beaumont Hospital
Dublin
Ireland

Sheila M Willatts MD FRCA FRCP
Consultant in Anaesthesia and Intensive Care
Bristol Royal Infirmary
United Bristol Healthcare NHS Trust
Bristol
United Kingdom

Jean-Louis Vincent MD PhD FCCM
Professor of Intensive Care and Head of Department
Department of Intensive Care
University Hospital Erasme
Brussels
Belgium

W. B. SAUNDERS

London • Edinburgh • New York • Philadelphia • St Louis • Sydney • Toronto • 2000

WB SAUNDERS
An imprint of Harcourt Publishers Limited

© Harcourt Publishers Limited 2000

Ⓧ is a registered trademark of Harcourt Publishers Limited

First published 2000

ISBN 0 7020 2242 X

British Library Cataloguing in Publication Data
A catalogue record for this book is available from the British Library

Library of Congress Cataloging in Publication Data
A catalog record for this book is available from the Library of Congress

Note
Medical knowledge is constantly changing. As new information becomes
available, changes in treatment, procedures, equipment and the use of drugs
become necessary. The authors and the publishers have taken care to ensure
that the information given in this text is accurate and up to date. However,
readers are strongly advised to confirm that the information, especially with
regard to drug usage, complies with the latest legislation and standards of
practice.

Printed in China

The
Publisher's
policy is to use
**paper manufactured
from sustainable forests**

Contents

Foreword

Despite the interest shown by the critical care community in the physiology of the response of the human organism to infection (sepsis), generally speaking, infections and infection control are not considered to be glamorous topics. However, a strong case could be made that the diagnosis, management and prevention of infections are crucial to the effective and efficient use of critical care resources. This volume is a valuable addition to the literature since it combines a discussion of sepsis and its mediators with a similarly broad discussion of individual infections and infection control issues in the intensive care unit.

At the turn of the new millennium it is almost impossible for anyone in the West to be unaware of the importance of infections. References to HIV/AIDS, hepatitis C, meningococcal meningitis, and the ravages of multi-resistant bacteria regularly appear in our news reports and on documentary programmes. The costs in human misery are considerable, as are the additional fiscal and societal costs of dealing with such infectious problems. It must be clear by now to most people, and certainly to physicians, that the earlier hope of controlling or eradicating infectious diseases is, for the most part, unjustifiable optimism. Apart from a few successes with viral diseases, our attempts to control infectious diseases, particularly those caused by bacteria, have been largely ineffective. Not only have we failed to make such diseases a thing of the past, but in fact, as a recent television documentary put it, "the bugs are fighting back". Bacterial infections are therefore of continuing, if not increasing, in importance to the general public, to all who practice medicine, and to those who practice critical care medicine in particular.

Not only are infections and infection control issues given relatively low prominence in the academic marketplace of the intensive care world, but worse yet, these are often subjects to which we play lip service in everyday practice. How often do we see even critical care physicians (let alone other physicians and health professionals) examine a patient without washing their hands before or after. How often do we maintain antibiotic treatment for prolonged periods even when there has been no evidence of a clinical response and no positive cultures have been reported. And how often do we then go on to broaden antibiotic cover, "just in case".

I accept that in the face of critical illness of uncertain aetiology, it is often difficult to know what is best, and that many decisions are, in the end, a judgement call. That being so, it is all the more important that we have available good information to guide (and hopefully refine) our decisions – that is the goal of evidence-based medicine, and infectious diseases in the critically ill is a topic which is certainly worthy of the evidence-based approach.

In that context, the authors of this volume have done us a good service (and one which is very timely) in pulling together a wealth of current information on infectious diseases in the critically ill. However, they have at the same time set themselves (or their successors) a major task for the future. Much of the material drawn together in this volume will change very rapidly, such is the level of research activity in areas such as cytokines and their antagonists, and apoptosis. It is to be hoped that we will soon have better diagnostic markers of sepsis, as well as better criteria for the diagnosis of important nosocomial problems in the critically ill patient such as ventilator-associated pneumonia, and line sepsis. It is also to be hoped that innovative approaches to the prevention and treatment of infections in the critically ill patient will be developed. If indeed all this does come about, the authors will have served us particularly well if they ensure that this text is regularly updated.

In the meantime, it is to be hoped that this volume gains the success it deserves as a scholarly condensation of many aspects of the literature available on the subject of infections in the critically ill.

Martin G. Tweeddale MBBS PhD FRCP
Clinical Director, Department of Intensive Care Medicine
Queen Alexandra Hospital, Portsmouth

Preface

In this book we have drawn together relevant information on the management of infection in the critically ill adult patient, especially those patients admitted to the intensive care unit (ICU). We have tried to emphasize the multidisciplinary nature of the approach to successful management, including the input of not just the intensivist and medical microbiologist or infectious-disease physician, but also that of the radiologist, surgeon and specialist physician as well as the invaluable contribution of nursing staff. For example, the opportunity to confirm a diagnosis may be lost for the absence of a telephone call to the medical microbiologist to find out the most appropriate specimen for investigation and diagnosis of a particular infection.

Whilst much of the approach outlined in this book reflects, we believe, optimal practice in the UK and Ireland, the principles should apply to most adult ICUs, wherever their location. However, local antimicrobial resistance patterns may preclude the use of some of the specific antimicrobial agents recommended. We would, in any event, encourage ICUs to draw up their own management and treatment policies as patient populations, facilities, expertise and staffing will vary from country to country and from unit to unit.

It is important for all those involved in the care of patients in the ICU to understand the pathogenesis and epidemiology of the various conditions discussed, as this will prompt appropriate investigations and the initiation of optimal empirical therapy. However, attention must also be given to preventing or minimizing infection, and one cannot exaggerate the importance of relatively cheap and simple but effective interventions such as washing hands after the examination of a patient, or ensuring the ICU is cleaned regularly.

In recent years great strides have been made in enhancing our understanding of the pathogenesis of ICU sepsis, but, as yet, this has not been translated into the routine use of novel therapeutic interventions such as monoclonal antibodies. Nonetheless, we have outlined in the first part of this book key aspects of the aetiology and pathogenesis of sepsis as well as epidemiology and prevention. This, we believe, will greatly enhance the usefulness of the second part of the book, which focuses on the major infections according to the organ systems. However, it should be stressed that infection in the critically ill is often polymicrobial and multi-organ in its aetiology and impact.

The references included represent further sources of information and evidence to justify recommendations, but these by no means represent the total literature on the subject. We have sought to ensure, where possible, that the guidance and recommendations provided are evidence based, but shared experience and common sense are important components in the successful management of infection. Finally, if – through the use of this book – we contribute in some way to improving the care of the infected ICU patient, then our labours will not have been in vain.

Hilary Humphreys
Sheila Willatts
Jean-Louis Vincent

January 2000

Acknowledgements

We are grateful to many colleagues, friends and members of our departments for their advice, guidance and assistance during the production of this work. In particular, we would like to thank Dr. Helen Enright, Dr. William Irving, Mr. Padraic Murray, Mr. Darragh Hynes, Dr. Donal Downey, Dr. Robert Spencer, Dr. Robert Winter, Professor David Speller and Dr. J. Virgee for their expert comments and helpful advice.

We also acknowledge the following for permission to include these illustrations: Dr. Donál Downey and the department of Diagnostic Radiology and Nuclear Medicine, University of Western Ontario, Canada (Figs 4.2–4.5, 7.1–7.4, 12.2), Professor Michael Lee (Figs 9.1 and 10.2), Dr. James Toland (Fig. 11.2), Dr. Erwin Brown (Plate 7) and Drs. Elaine Kay and Antoinette Grace (Plates 6 and 12).

Abbreviations

AIDS	acquired immune deficiency syndrome
APACHE	Acute Physiology and Chronic Health Evaluation
ARDS	acute respiratory distress syndrome
ATLS	advanced trauma life support
BAL	bronchoalveolar lavage
BHSA	β-haemolytic streptococcus group A
BNF	British National Formulary
BP	blood pressure
BPI	bactericidal permeability-increasing protein
cAMP	cyclic adenosine monophosphate
CAPD	continuous ambulatory peritoneal dialysis
CARS	counter anti-inflammatory response syndrome
CDC	Centers for Disease Control and Prevention
CFU	colony forming unit
cGMP	cyclic guanosine monophosphate
CHAOS	cardiovascular compromise and shock, homeostasis, apoptosis, organ dysfunction, suppression of the immune system
CJD	Creutzfeldt–Jakob disease
CMV	cytomegalovirus
cNOS	constitutive nitric oxide synthase
CNS	central nervous system
COPD	chronic obstructive pulmonary disease
CRP	C-reactive protein
CSF	cerebrospinal fluid
CSU	catheter specimen of urine
CT	computed tomography
CVC	central venous catheter
CVP	central venous pressure
DEAFF	detection of early antigen fluorescent foci
DIC	disseminated intravascular coagulation
Do_2	oxygen delivery
ECG	electrocardiogram
EEG	electroencephalogram
EIA	enzyme immunoassay
EPIC	European Prevalence of Infection in Intensive Care Study
ERCP	endoscopic retrograde cholangiopancreatography
ESR	erythrocyte sedimentation rate
EVD	external ventricular drain
Flo_2	inspired oxygen fraction
G-CSF	granulocyte colony-stimulating factor
HAART	highly active anti-retroviral therapy

HBV	hepatitis B virus
HCV	hepatitis C virus
HCW	health care worker
HIV	human immunodeficiency virus
HSE	herpes simplex encephalitis
HSV	herpes simplex virus
HTIG	human tetanus immunoglobulin
ICAM	intercellular adhesion molecule
ICP	intracranial pressure
ICU	intensive care unit
Ig	immunoglobulin
IL	interleukin
IL-1ra	interleukin 1 receptor antagonist
iNOS	inducible nitric oxide synthase
L-NAME	L-N-arginine methyl ester
L-NMMA	L-N-monomethyl-arginine
LP	lumbar puncture
LPS	lipopolysaccharide
MARS	mixed anti-inflammatory response syndrome
MHC	major histocompatibility complex
MOF	multi-organ failure
MRI	magnetic resonance imaging
MRSA	methicillin-resistant *Staphylococcus aureus*
NAC	N-acetyl-L-cysteine
NF	nuclear factor
NO	nitric oxide
NOS	nitric oxide synthase
OHD	occupational health department
OPSI	overwhelming post-splenectomy infection
PAF	platelet-activating factor
Pao_2	arterial oxygen pressure
PBS	protected brush or catheter specimen
PCR	polymerase chain reaction
pHi	intramucosal pH
PLA_2	phospholipase A_2
PUO	pyrexia of unknown origin
SDD	selective decontamination of the digestive tract
SIRS	systemic inflammatory response syndrome
Svo_2	mixed venous oxygen saturation
SVR	systemic vascular resistance
TB	tuberculosis
TGF	transforming growth factor
T_H	T helper cell
TNF	tumour necrosis factor
TOE	transoesophageal echocardiography

TPN	total parenteral nutrition
TTE	transthoracic echocardiography
US	ultrasonography
UTI	urinary tract infection
vCJD	variant Creutzfeldt–Jakob disease
VDRL	venereal disease reference laboratory
Vo_2	oxygen uptake
VRE	vancomycin-resistant enterococci
VZV	varicella-zoster virus
WBC	white blood cell

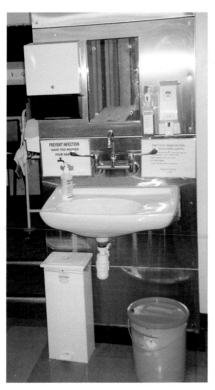

Plate 1 Hand-washing facilities including elbow-operated taps, soap/disinfectant dispenser, paper-towels and foot-operated bin.

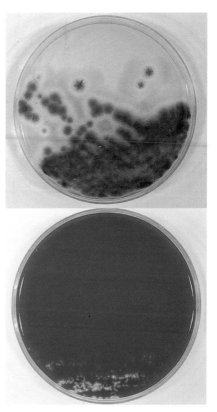

Plate 3 Heavy growth of *Aspergillus* spp. on Saboraud agar (A) compared with blood agar (B).

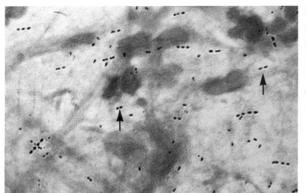

Plate 2 Gram stain of purulent sputum as indicated by the presence of 'pus' cells. Numerous Gram-positive diplococci are present (arrows).

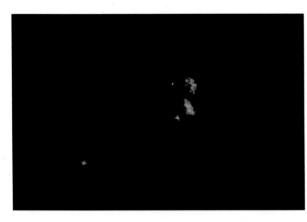

Plate 4 Diagnosis of influenza A confirmed by antigen detection in bronchoalveolar lavage specimen using specific fluorescent antibodies.

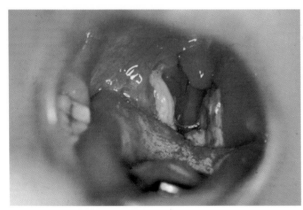

Plate 5 Tonsillar membrane characteristic of diphtheria. (Courtesy of Dr I. Zamiri; published in Emond RTD *et al*. (1995) *Colour Atlas of Infectious Diseases*, 3rd edit. Mosby-Wolfe: London.)

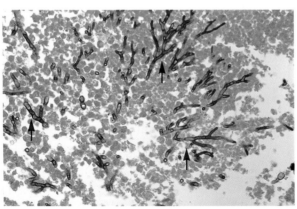

Plate 6 Histological section of lung tissue (Grocot stain) demonstrating hyphae (arrows) indicative of invasive aspergillosis.

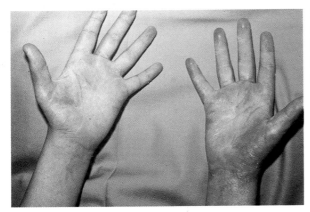

Plate 7 Desquamation of the palms of the hands, one of the later manifestations of toxic shock syndrome.

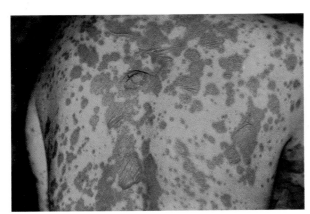

Plate 8 Toxic epidermal necrolysis. (Courtesy of Emond RTD *et al.* (1995) *Colour Atlas of Infectious Diseases*, 3rd edit. Mosby-Wolfe: London.)

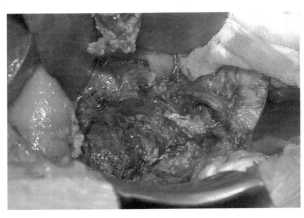

Plate 9 Operative view of necrotizing pancreatitis.

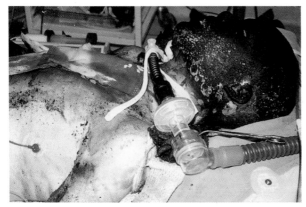

Plate 10 Extensive burns with fasciotomy.

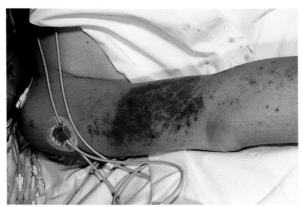

Plate 11 Purpuric rash.

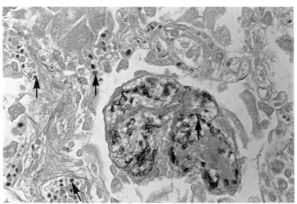

Plate 12 Diagnosis of *P. carinii*. Histological section of lung tissue (Grocott stain) showing *P. carinii* cysts (arrows) indicative of infection.

Section 1

General Background

1 Pathogenesis of infection in the intensive care unit

INTRODUCTION

Patients requiring intensive therapy are very susceptible to infection due to acquired defects in host defence mechanisms from the immunosuppressive effects of anaesthesia, surgery and drug therapy, the use of invasive monitoring techniques and the severity of the underlying illness requiring admission. The use of broad-spectrum antibiotics, which alter normal bacterial flora, may predispose to infection with resistant organisms; nosocomial infection delays patient discharge from the intensive care unit (ICU) and from hospital, and contributes significantly to morbidity[1, 2].

INCIDENCE AND AETIOLOGY

Infection occurs in 15–40% of all ICU admissions and the crude mortality rate is between 10 and 80% but this includes mortality from the underlying condition[3]. A European study (EPIC) of the prevalence of infection reviewed 10,038 patients and found that 45% were infected and 21% had acquired their infection in the intensive care unit (ICU). Pneumonia (47%), lower respiratory tract infection (18%), urinary tract infection (17%) and blood stream infection (12%) were the most frequent types of infection reported. The most frequently reported organisms were Enterbacteriaceae (34%), *Staphylococcus aureus* (30%, of which 60% were resistant to methicillin) and *Pseudomonas aeruginosa* (29%). Seven risk factors for ICU-acquired infection were identified: length of stay longer than 48 hours, mechanical ventilation, a diagnosis of trauma, central venous, pulmonary artery and urinary catheterisation and stress ulcer prophylaxis[3]. The highest infection rates are seen in surgical, burns, trauma and neonatal ICUs[4]. Patients in the ICU rapidly become colonized with potentially pathogenic Gram-negative bacilli, Gram-positive cocci and *Candida* spp. The prevalence of these colonizing organisms is not decreased by parenteral broad-spectrum antibiotics but is reduced in the gastrointestinal tract by selective decontamination of the digestive tract (SDD)[5]. However, the overuse of parenteral broad-spectrum antibiotics in ICUs results in the infections acquired by patients in ICUs being resistant to first-line antimicrobial agents more often than infections acquired elsewhere in the hospital[1].

In the USA, 10–15% of patients arrive at hospital with a clinically significant infection or develop one at some point during their hospital stay. Half are due to

Gram-negative organisms, and of these 10–20% may result in bacteraemia with attendant haemodynamic instability and organ dysfunction[3, 6–9]. Risk factors for the development of pneumonia include coma, trauma, the need for respiratory support, an Acute Physiology and Chronic Health Evaluation (APACHE) II score greater than 16 and impaired airway reflexes on admission[3, 10]. The epidemiology of infection in the ICU is discussed in greater detail in Chapter 2.

UNDERLYING CONCEPTS

Sepsis and the systemic inflammatory response syndrome

With the development of the concept of the systemic inflammatory response syndrome (SIRS), attempts have been made to standardize diagnostic criteria for sepsis, severe sepsis and septic shock[11, 12]. A positive blood culture confirms infection but less than 50% of patients with sepsis will have laboratory-confirmed bacteraemia. Whilst the term 'sepsis' was equated with microbial infection in the past, it is now clear that this is also an immunological response to a variety of insults such as a major burn or pancreatitis. The presence of bacteria is not necessary for the development of sepsis as endotoxin alone can precipitate a cascade of mediators often leading to septic shock, with tissue hypoxia and subsequent multiple organ failure. Sepsis can therefore be defined as the systemic response to infection induced either by the presence of pathogenic microbial agents in the bloodstream or by the release of toxic products from a focal infection or in response to non-infective conditions such as trauma, pancreatitis and following cardiopulmonary bypass. SIRS is therefore a non-specific term and should not be applied in the absence of a full clinical assessment (Table 1.1). There are now good data relating to the evolution of SIRS into septic shock and multiple organ failure[13, 14].

Septic shock

Patients with septic shock are those with hypotension despite adequate fluid resuscitation and with evidence of perfusion abnormalities such as lactic acidosis, oliguria or an acute alteration in mental status. Patients receiving inotropic or vasopressor agents may not be hypotensive at the time that perfusion abnormalities are measured and are therefore excluded from the definition.

The cause of sepsis in 'clean' cases of trauma is probably the translocation of bacteria across the wall of hypoperfused gut during the initial period of shock. Subsequent or concurrent release of endotoxin and its associated mediators leads to peripheral ischaemia and progressive multi-organ failure (MOF). This ischaemia occurs in the face of often supranormal oxygen delivery, but oxygen demand is increased and extraction is impaired[7, 15].

We now understand a great deal more about sepsis, particularly the under-lying biochemical and cellular processes involved[16], and we also appreciate that the clinical manifestations of sepsis may develop without documented infection. SIRS, which reflects common pathogenic pathways, is therefore increasingly used as an all-encompassing term.

Table 1.1 Definitions[11, 12].

Infection	An inflammatory response induced by the presence of pathogenic micro-organisms, or the invasion of normally sterile host tissue by microbial pathogens
Bacteraemia	The presence of bacteria in the bloodstream; laboratory confirmation will depend on the amount of blood cultured and the sensitivity of methods used in the laboratory
Sepsis/SIRS	SIRS is characterized by two or more of the following: • core temperature $<36°C$ or $>39°C$ • tachycardia defined as heart rate >90 beats/min in the absence of β-blocking drugs • tachypnoea defined as respiratory rate >20 breaths/min or $Paco_2$ <4.3 kPa (32 mmHg) during spontaneous ventilation or the requirement for mechanical ventilation • white blood cell count >12 or $<3 \times 10^9$ l^{-1} or $>10\%$ immature (band) form
Severe sepsis	A clinical suspicion of infection requiring the initiation or change of systemic antimicrobial therapy within the last 72 hours and a systemic inflammatory response and acute onset of end-organ dysfunction in the preceding 24 hours unrelated to the primary focus of infection and not explained by any chronic underlying disease
Septic shock	Arterial hypotension (systolic arterial blood pressure (BP) <90 mmHg or mean arterial BP <60 mmHg or a reduction of >40 mmHg from baseline in the absence of other causes for hypotension) with associated signs of tissue hypoperfusion Increased blood lactate >2 mmol l^{-1}

Effects on organ function

Acute and chronic sequelae of the sepsis syndrome are the thirteenth leading cause of death in the USA[17, 18]. Death due to MOF is now more common than death due to circulatory failure following improvements in cardiovascular support. The mortality from sepsis varies with the extent of organ failure. When three systems are in failure for 3 or more days, the outcome is very poor, even in young, previously fit adults[19]. The overall mortality rate from sepsis is 20–60% and, using the definitions in Table 1.1, mortality rate can be predicted: 7% for SIRS and up to 45% for septic shock[20]. It is believed that new therapies

(Chapter 6) benefit some patients even if no effect on overall mortality has been demonstrated; consequently, severity scoring and risk prediction models are a key part of future research and clinical studies.

Based on Newtonian principles of equal and opposite counter-effects for all reactions, Bone developed the concept of innate anti-inflammatory activity which may affect prognosis[21]. This is helpful in understanding the pathophysiology of sepsis and the variable patient response. The basis of this concept is that an initial insult (bacterial, viral, traumatic or thermal) will initiate both a local pro-inflammatory response and a local anti-inflammatory response. The mediators produced by both pro- and anti-inflammatory responses will spill over into the circulation producing a systemic reaction. This may be predominantly pro-inflammatory (SIRS) or a counter anti-inflammatory response syndrome (CARS) or a mixture of the two (mixed anti-inflammatory response syndrome; MARS). CHAOS results from a series of effects: Cardiovascular compromise and shock where SIRS predominates, Homeostasis where CARS and SIRS are balanced, Apoptosis or cell death, Organ dysfunction where SIRS predominates in both conditions and Suppression of the immune system where CARS predominates. The outcome of the septic episode will depend upon the balance of these mechanisms[21]. What is clear is that development of MOF has a poor prognosis and this may be predicted by serial estimation of blood lactate levels[22].

Organ dysfunction begins in the acutely ill patient with SIRS when homeostasis cannot be maintained without intervention[23]. The commonest organ to be affected is the lung with development of acute lung injury (Pao_2 (mmHg)/Fio_2 <300), and then, as the condition worsens, acute respiratory distress syndrome (ARDS; Pao_2 (mmHg)/Fio_2 <200). ARDS occurs in about 28% of these patients but hepatic, renal and other organ failure rapidly follow

Table 1.2 Changes induced by the 'cytokine cascade'.

Thermoregulation
Vascular permeability
Vascular tone
Myocardial depression
Bone marrow function
Activity of key enzymes
Stimulation of further mediators
  PAF
  Eicosanoids
  Other cascade activation
    Complement
    Kinins
    Coagulation
    Other interleukins
  Transforming growth factor β
  Prostaglandin E

with the development of disseminated intravascular coagulation (DIC), gastro-intestinal stress ulceration and failure to absorb nutrients.

Diagnostic criteria for organ failure were produced by the Consensus Conference of the American Conference of Chest Physicians and the Society for Critical Care Medicine in 1992 and are summarized in Table 1.1. However, it is increasingly recognized that a continuum of dysfunction occurs and a graded score should be used; several of these are under development[24, 25, 26].

CLINICAL FEATURES OF SEPSIS

Clearer definitions have facilitated the management of individual patients and enabled comparative trials of new anti-infective agents to be undertaken. Sepsis is characterized by the following clinical features: fever, tachypnoea which often results in respiratory alkalosis, and tachycardia. There is usually an increased cardiac output and a low systemic vascular resistance (SVR). There may be either a leukocytosis (+ left shift) or leukopenia (Table 1.1). These features are accompanied by an increase in cellular metabolism, increased oxygen consumption and increased insulin requirements initially, but often hypoglycaemia occurs at a later stage. Cutaneous manifestations such as purpura are less common.

Laboratory indicators of inflammation include increased erythrocyte sedimentation rate (ESR), viscosity, C-reactive protein and fibrinogen levels, with increased cytokine concentration, particularly tumour necrosis factor (TNF) and interleukins (see below). Other markers that may be used but are often not available routinely include elastase, neopterin and procalcitonin. As the condition develops, organ dysfunction worsens.

However, few of the above clinical or laboratory features are specific for sepsis. Fever may arise from autonomic dysfunction after cerebral insults; autonomic dysfunction is associated with increased oxygen consumption and worsening cerebral ischaemia and many of the cytokines such as TNF and interleukin 1 (IL-1) are capable of inducing fever in their own right.

THE CYTOKINE RESPONSE TO SEPSIS

Micro-organisms or their cell wall products such as endotoxin (Gram-negative bacteria) or teichoic acid (Gram-positive bacteria) stimulate the production of inflammatory mediators such as cytokines, which have multiple and often cumulative effects[27, 28]. Cytokines are soluble molecules, usually proteins, that allow for communication between cells and regulate the amplitude and duration of immune and inflammatory responses. Their specific actions depend upon the stimulus, the receptor cell type and the presence of other mediators and they include low molecular weight protein and lipid mediators[28]. The biological activity of cytokines (Table 1.2) is regulated by specific cellular receptors which may be membrane bound or shed into the circulation. These receptors constitute a natural regulatory mechanism to limit the deleterious effect of overstimulation. In particular, TNFα and IL-1 are key mediators in sepsis.

Because cytokines are paracrine agents, i.e. locally active on a variety of tissues at their site of production, it is difficult to correlate the plasma concentration of a particular pro-inflammatory cytokine with the extent of the tissue damage it may cause. Cytokines are not stored but newly synthesized and released in response to inflammatory stimuli by gene transcription with new expression of the cytokine messenger RNA. Each cytokine has a variety of transcription factor binding domains which interact in a complex way. One transcription factor – nuclear factor NF-κB – appears to play a central role in regulating the cytokine cascade and is activated in many cell types by stimuli such as endotoxin, TNFα and IL-1 (Figure 1.1).

The mediator network consists of the interaction of cytokines, adhesion molecules, arachidonic acid metabolites, platelet-activating factor (PAF), oxygen free radicals, nitric oxide and other mediators, all of which induce hypotension, myocardial depression, capillary leak and inflammation. There is increased oxygen demand, fever and hypermetabolism, and oxygen consumption may be limited by the circulatory changes, resulting in tissue hypoxia.

Secondary mediators include lipids, prostaglandin I_2, thromboxane A_2, endorphins, peptides including vasoactive intestinal peptide, amines, histamine and serotonin. The central pro-inflammatory role of IL-1 and TNF in septic shock is related to their ability to activate endothelial cells, induce the production of other inflammatory cytokines (IL-8, IL-6 and colony stimulating factor), activate effector cells (T and B lymphocytes, monocytes, macrophages and neutrophils) and release PAF and other downstream mediators, including anti-inflammatory cytokines.

Tumour necrosis factor α

TNFα is a 17 kDa protein produced primarily by mononuclear phagocytes. Infusion of TNFα in humans produces SIRS with fever, haemodynamic disturbance, leukopenia, elevated liver enzymes and coagulopathy. TNF increases neutrophil margination, activates the antimicrobial action of monocytes, macrophages and neutrophils, induces the non-specific acute-phase protein response with fever and anorexia, increases muscle degradation for gluconeogenesis and provides substrates for increased visceral protein synthesis. At wound sites, TNF increases vascular proliferation, osteoclastic activity and collagen synthesis allowing remodelling of the wound area. It is a potent inducer of other cytokines. Plasma concentrations generally correlate with the severity of sepsis and outcome and a persistent increase in TNF levels is associated with a poor prognosis[27].

Although TNF is released mainly from macrophages during sepsis, other sources include the lung, pancreas, heart, spleen, kidney, uterus and fallopian tubes. It is also an important mediator in haemorrhagic shock, trauma and burn injury, end-stage heart failure, acute liver failure, rheumatoid arthritis, allograft rejection and some forms of cancer.

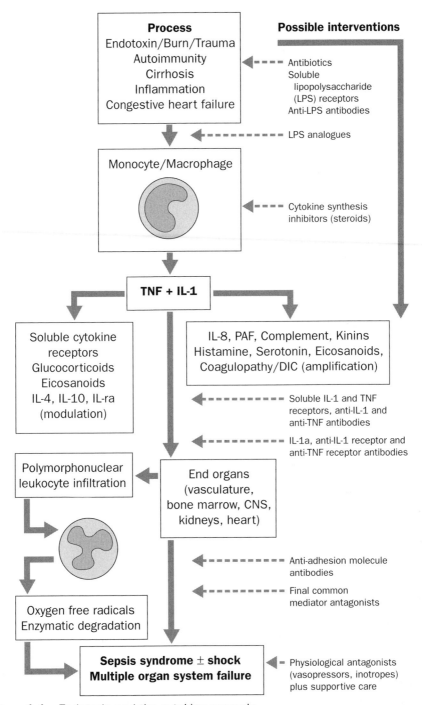

Figure 1.1 Endotoxin and the cytokine cascade.

Interleukin 1

IL-1 is a strong immune adjuvant that increases cellular antimicrobial activity and initiates the pro-inflammatory cascade, including a rapid increase in IL-6 levels. There are two related proteins, IL-1α and IL-1β, which activate the same IL-1 receptors and share the same biological activity. Both are produced by mononuclear phagocytes and polymorphonuclear leukocytes, and mimic the effects of TNF. IL-1β activates the production of IL-6, IL-8 and TNF, and appears to correlate with the severity of sepsis but is detectable in only a minority of patients.

Interleukin 6

IL-6 is a 21 kDa glycoprotein which activates B and T lymphocytes, induces acute-phase protein production, modulates haematopoiesis, activates the coagulation system and causes fever. After experimental injection of endotoxin in animals, plasma IL-6 is detectable later than the maximal concentrations of TNF and IL-1. Although there is no statistically significant relationship between endotoxin concentration and mortality, there is a strong association between IL-6 and mortality[29]. In animals, blocking IL-6 does not improve outcome but endotoxin-induced activation of coagulation is attenuated. The role of IL-6 in inflammation is not clearly defined but it does seem to correlate more closely than other cytokines with the severity and outcome of human sepsis. In patients with suspected acute sepsis, plasma IL-6 concentration predicts bacteraemia and subsequent death from infection.

Other cytokines

IL-8 is a small protein produced by a variety of cells and released in response to endotoxin and TNF. Local release of IL-8 recruits and activates neutrophils resulting in tissue damage and organ dysfunction. It also attracts basophils and T lymphocytes and has been implicated as an angiogenic factor. IL-8 may be important in mediating ARDS.

IL-10 is produced by T helper lymphocytes and inhibits cytokine production by activated macrophages, thus expressing counter-inflammatory properties. In animal models it protects against a lethal dose of endotoxin. IL-10 is detected in the plasma of patients with septic shock in higher concentrations than in those with sepsis alone.

Adhesion molecules

Adhesion molecules are important facilitators of endothelial cell–leukocyte interactions. A series of integrins (CD11, CD18) bind to members of the immunoglobulin supergene family, including intercellular adhesion molecule (ICAM) 1 and 2.

Other mediators

As with all inflammatory processes, oxygen free radicals have an important role. Bacterial endotoxin and other cytokines induce expression of inducible nitric oxide synthase in many tissues. The nitric oxide released results in profound vasodilatation, vascular permeability and circulatory failure (see below). PAF probably acts by priming and amplifying inflammatory mediator release, initially $TNF\alpha$ and later thromboxane A_2 and leukotriene B_4.

THE ANTIBODY AND CELLULAR IMMUNE RESPONSE TO INFECTION

The immune defences against infection include non-specific or innate defences and the specific immune response. The innate defences include the skin, mucous secretion, gastric acid and complement activation. When these defences are overcome, organisms are killed by lysosomes and phagocytosis. The cells involved in this include phagocytes (polymorphs, macrophages, mast cells), endothelial cells and hepatocytes. Cells infected with viruses and parasites are killed by large granular lymphocytes (natural killer cells) and eosinophils. Innate immunity provides rapid, incomplete, antimicrobial host defence until the slower, more specific acquired immune response develops. However, innate immunity may have an additional role in determining which antigens the acquired immune system responds to, and the nature of that response.

T and B lymphocyte responses
Immunity to some pathogens is acquired by antibodies that activate complement, stimulate phagocytes and specifically inactivate micro-organisms not destroyed by innate immunity. Lymphocytes are the basis of the acquired immune system, as are antibody-producing plasma cells derived from T and B lymphocytes. T and B lymphocyte function is impaired in critical illness leading to a relatively immunocompromised state, increased susceptibility to infection and reduced ability to control infection when it does occur.

Both T and B lymphocytes are involved in developing the immune response to infection; production of antibody is the main function of B cells, with T cells being important for resisting intracellular organisms. Rarely, however, do T and B cells act independently. T cells are divided into two subsets, $CD4^+$ and $CD8^+$, on the basis of receptor surface molecules (Figure 1.2). Generally speaking, $CD4^+$ T cells have helper functions in augmenting T and B cell proliferation and activation[16]. $CD4^+$ T cells, via the cytokines they produce, play a pivotal role in the induction and regulation of cell-mediated and humoral immunity. Protective responses to pathogens are dependent on activation of the appropriate T helper cell subset accompanied by a characteristic set of immune effector functions. Evidence to date suggests that cytokines produced by helper cells are important regulators of lymphocyte subset activation and differentiation. Micro-organisms bind to antibodies on the surface of B cells such that subsequent responses are faster and amplified. T cells secrete soluble mediators which activate other cells to enhance microbial defence mechanisms and produce cytolytic T cells which kill target organisms.

The major histocompatibility complex (MHC) includes genes encoding class I and II cell surface glycoproteins whose function is to present antigen peptides

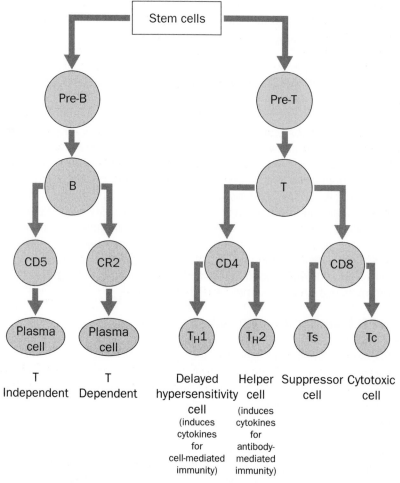

Figure 1.2 Origin and classification of lymphocytes.

to T cells. Regulation of MHC gene expression plays a fundamental role in the immune system because alteration of cell surface expression of class I or II molecules can affect the efficiency of antigen presentation. T helper cells recognize class II MHC molecules and produce interferon γ and other macrophage-activating factors. Cytotoxic or killer T cells recognize specific antigens and class I MHC molecules on the surface of infected cells.

THERAPEUTIC IMPLICATIONS

Non-specific immunostimulation has progressed from crude microbially derived substances to chemically defined drugs with selective effects on different components of the immune system. Hybridoma technology has facilitated the production of rodent monoclonal antibodies against human pathogens and cells, but these have limited clinical application. Protein engineering is now generating antibodies for treatment of infectious diseases, autoimmune diseases and cancer by 'humanizing' rodent antibodies. Humanized antibodies have improved pharmacokinetics, reduced immunogenicity and have been used to some clinical advantage.

The first approach to immune manipulation was treatment with very large doses of steroids until it became clear that this approach had little effect[30]. It then seemed logical to target some of the other toxins released from bacteria for neutralization. This was the concept behind the development of monoclonal antibodies against the lipid A core of endotoxin common to all Gram-negative organisms (Chapter 6). This approach has, however, been disappointing and has largely been abandoned.

Soluble cytokine receptors and receptor antagonists

Soluble cytokine receptors have been described for TNFα, IL-1β and IL-6. TNF receptors are produced by proteolytic cleavage of the extracellular binding domain of the TNF receptor on the surface of the cell. Surface TNF receptors are present in normal humans and are released in response to endotoxin, peaking 1 hour after exposure. Plasma concentration of these receptors correlates with mortality. The receptor for IL-1 is a 23 kDa molecule which attenuates endotoxin effects in animals. It should therefore be theoretically possible to modulate the cytokine response to infection by the administration of such receptor antagonists.

Nitric oxide

The L-arginine/nitric oxide (NO) pathway is involved in many cardiovascular and CNS physiological processes where NO is generated by constitutive nitric oxide synthase (cNOS), requiring increased intracellular calcium levels for activation[31]. Nitric oxide may be the common mechanism by which microbial products and cytokines have their deleterious action on the cardiovascular system[32]. Analogues of L-arginine such as L-N-monomethyl-arginine (L-NMMA) inhibit the production of NO by combining with the substrate binding site of inducible nitric oxide synthase (iNOS). The resultant decrease in NO leads to reduced synthesis of cyclic guanosine monophosphate (cGMP) and vasoconstriction[33].

Endothelial cNOS may also be important for maintaining vascular permeability and integrity. Inhibition of cNOS increases microvascular fluid and protein flux. Endotoxin and inflammatory mediators such as PAF rapidly increase intestinal vascular permeability, which can be modified by pretreatment with cNOS inhibitors and enhanced by concomitant administration of NO donors[32]. Nitric oxide generated by the coronary vessels increases coronary blood flow and myocardial supply, and that generated by the endocardium may have a negative inotropic effect on the heart contractility.

Inhibitors of iNOS may be of benefit in sepsis by restoring cardiovascular homeostasis. These inhibitors fall into two categories:

1. Inhibitors of the expression of NOS (glucocorticoids). Dexamethasone inhibits the decrease in vascular tone, the rise in cGMP levels and the induction of calcium-independent NOS, without affecting cNOS.
2. Inhibitors of the activity of NOS (L-NMMA, methylene blue). Methylene blue reduces NO generation and activation by inhibition of NOS and soluble guanylate cyclase through interaction with the haem moiety of these enzymes, as well as by direct inactivation of NO through its redox properties.

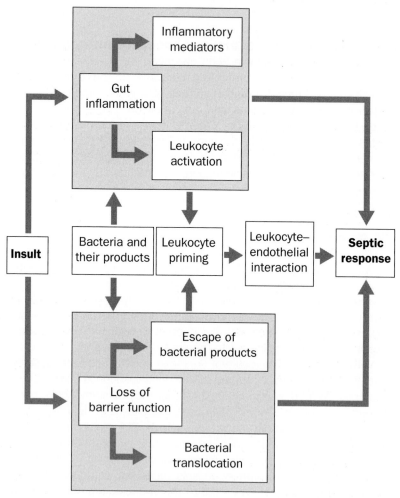

Figure 1.3   Initiation of a septic response.

MANAGEMENT

Despite an increased understanding of the pathophysiology of sepsis (Figure 1.3), there have to date been very few anti-inflammatory agents that have proven to have any significant clinical benefit in the management of severe sepsis and SIRS[29, 34-36]. This will, however, be discussed in Chapter 6. Treatment remains supportive. Administration of antipyretic agents is controversial; on one hand they be beneficial by reducing oxygen consumption in some circumstances, such as cerebral oedema, but on the other they may be disadvantageous, perhaps by reducing production of heat shock proteins.

Key points

- Patients requiring intensive care are highly susceptible to infection due to the immunosuppressive effects of drugs and disease.
- Nosocomial infection delays discharge from the ICU and contributes to mortality.
- Septic shock leads to multiple organ failure and death.
- Endotoxin initiates an inflammatory cytokine cascade, a complex pathophysiological system of chemical and cellular events.
- Management is supportive as very few new agents provide specific benefit.

REFERENCES

1. Solomkin JS (1996) Antimicrobial resistance: an overview. *New Horizons* **4**: 319–320.
2. Expert Report of the European Society of Intensive Care Medicine (1994) The problem of sepsis. *Intensive Care Medicine* **20**: 300–304.
3. Vincent J-L, Bihari D, Suter P et al. (1995) The prevalence of nosocomial infection in intensive care units in Europe. Results of the European Prevalence of Infection in Intensive Care (EPIC) Study. EPIC International Advisory Committee. *Journal of the American Medical Association* **274**: 639–644.
4. Pittet D, Rangel-Frausto MS, Li N et al. (1995) Systemic inflammatory response syndrome, sepsis, severe sepsis and septic shock: incidence, morbidities and outcomes in surgical patients. *Intensive Care Medicine* **21**: 302–309.
5. D'Amico R, Pifferi S, Leonetti C et al. (1998) Effectiveness of antibiotic prophylaxis in critically ill adult patients: systematic review of randomized controlled trials. *British Medical Journal* **316**: 1275–1285.
6. Bone RC, Fisher CJ, Clemmer TP et al. (1989) Sepsis syndrome: a valid clinical entity. *Critical Care Medicine* **17**: 389–393.
7. Hayes MA, Yau EHS, Timmins AC et al. (1993) Response of critically ill patients to treatment aimed at achieving supranormal oxygen delivery and consumption. *Chest* **103**: 886–895.

8. Kreger BE, Craven DE, McCabe WR (1980) Gram-negative bacteremia IV. Re-evaluation of clinical features and treatment in 612 patients. *American Journal of Medicine* **63**: 344–355.

9. Parker MM, Parillo JE (1983) Septic shock: hemodynamics and pathogenesis. *Journal of the American Medical Association* **250**: 3324.

10. Chevret S, Hemmer M, Carlet J et al. (1993) Incidence and risk factors of pneumonia acquired in intensive care units: results from a multicentre prospective study on 996 patients. *Intensive Care Medicine* **19**: 256–264.

11. American College of Chest Physicians/Society of Critical Care Medicine Consensus Conference (1992) Definition for sepsis and organ failure and guidelines for the use of innovative therapy in sepsis. *Chest* **20**: 864–874.

12. Centers for Disease Control (1989) Definitions for nosocomial infections (1988–1989). *American Review of Respiratory Disease* **139**: 1058–1059.

13. Salvo I, de Clan W, Mussico M et al. (1995) The Italian SEPSIS study: preliminary results of the incidence and evolution of SIRS, sepsis, severe sepsis and septic shock. *Intensive Care Medicine* **21**: S244–S249.

14. Smail N, Messiah A, Edouard A et al. (1995) Role of systemic inflammatory response syndrome and infection in the occurrence of early multiple organ dysfunction syndrome following severe trauma. *Intensive Care Medicine* **21**: 813–816.

15. Shoemaker WC, Appel PL, Kram HB (1992) Role of oxygen debt in the development of organ failure, sepsis and death in high-risk surgical patients. *Chest* **102**: 208–215.

16. Abraham E (1993) Sepsis: cellular and physiological mechanisms. *New Horizons* **1**: 1–83.

17. Machiedo GW, Loverme PJ, McGovern PJ et al. (1981) Patterns of mortality in surgical intensive care units. *Surgery, Gynecology and Obstetrics* **152**: 757–759.

18. Kreger BE, Craven DE, Carling PC et al. (1980) Gram-negative bacteremia III. Reassessment of etiology, epidemiology and ecology in 612 patients. *American Journal of Medicine* **63**: 332–343.

19. Knaus WA, Draper EA, Wagner DP et al. (1985) Prognosis in acute organ failure. *Annals of Surgery* **202**: 685–693.

20. Rangel-Frausto MS, Pittet D, Costigan M et al. (1995) The natural history of the systemic inflammatory response syndrome (SIRS): a prospective study. *Journal of the American Medical Association* **11**: 117–123.

21. Bone RC (1996) Sir Isaac Newton, sepsis, SIRS and CARS. *Critical Care Medicine* **24**: 1125–1128.

22. Bakker J, Gris P, Coffernils M et al. (1996) Serial blood lactate levels can predict the development of multiple organ failure following septic shock. *American Journal of Surgery* **171**: 221–226.

23. Deitch EA (1992) Multiple organ failure. *Annals of Surgery* **216**: 117–134.

24. Marshall JC, Cook DJ, Christou NV et al. (1995) The multiple organ dysfunction (MOD) score: a reliable descriptor of a complex clinical outcome. *Critical Care Medicine* **23**: 1638–1652.

25. Le Gall J-R, Klar J, Lemeshow S et al. (1996) The logistic organ dysfunction system. A new way to assess organ dysfunction in the intensive care unit. *Journal of the American Medical Association* **276**: 802–810.

26. Vincent J-L, de Mendonca A, Cantraune F et al. (1998) Use of the SOFA score to assess the incidence of organ system dysfunction/failure in intensive care units: results of a multi-center, prospective study. *Critical Care Medicine* **26**: 1793–1800.

27. Blackwell TS, Christman JW (1996) Sepsis and cytokines: current status. *British Journal of Anaesthesia* **77**: 110–117.
28. Galley HF, Webster NR (1996) The immuno-inflammatory cascade. *British Journal of Anaesthesia* **77**: 11–16.
29. RAMSES Study (1998) Treatment of severe sepsis in patients with highly inflated IL-6 levels with anti-TNF monoclonal antibody-fragment Afelimomal (MAK 195F): the RAMSES study. (Abstract) *Critical Care* **2** (Suppl 1): 18.
30. Lefering R, Neugebauer EAM (1995) Steroid controversy in sepsis and septic shock: a meta-analysis. *Critical Care Medicine* **23**: 1294–1303.
31. Moncado S, Palmer RM, Higgs EA (1992) Nitric oxide physiology, pathophysiology and pharmacology. *Pharmacological Reviews* **43**: 109–142.
32. Rees DD (1995) Role of nitric oxide in the vascular dysfunction of septic shock. *Biochemical Society Transactions* **23**: 1025–1029.
33. Whittle BJR (1994) Nitric oxide in physiology and pathology. *Histochemical Journal* **27**: 727–737.
34. Giroir BP (1993) Mediators of septic shock. New approaches for interrupting the endogenous inflammatory cascade. *Critical Care Medicine* **21**: 780–789.
35. Eidelman LA, Sprung CL (1994) Why have new effective therapies for sepsis not been developed? *Critical Care Medicine* **22**: 1330–1334.
36. Shapiro L, Gelfand JA (1993) Cytokines and sepsis: pathophysiology and therapy. *New Horizons* **1**: 13–22.

2   Epidemiology of infection

CLASSIFICATION

Infection in the intensive care unit (ICU) may be community, hospital or ICU acquired. Hospital and ICU-acquired infections are those not present on admission to the hospital or unit, respectively. In practice, this usually means that an infection apparent 48 hours or more after admission was not acquired in the community. Exceptions to this occur when the incubation period is relatively long, e.g. legionnaires' disease and typhoid fever. These distinctions, although somewhat arbitrary, are helpful in predicting the likely pathogens causing infection in the ICU and when devising empirical antimicrobial treatment regimens.

Infection may also be classified as endogenous, i.e. infection caused by microbes that are part of the patient's own flora (e.g. surgical peritonitis), or exogenous, i.e. infection caused by microbes acquired from the environment or from other patients (e.g. cross-infection with *Pseudomonas aeruginosa*). In practice, it is often difficult to distinguish between the two in the absence of intense surveillance and sophisticated laboratory techniques to characterize and type bacteria. Furthermore, this categorization does not take account of the variation in patients' flora which occurs following admission to the ICU, and the complex interaction between patients, staff and the environment in the ICU, which can be fully understood only with the help of continuous surveillance[1]. This, however is not always practicable, or financially feasible.

PREVALENCE AND RISK FACTORS

The frequency of hospital-acquired (nosocomial) infection is especially high in the ICU compared with other clinical areas of the hospital. In a recent prevalence survey of infection in hospitals conducted throughout the UK and Ireland, 15% of patients had community-acquired infection with 9% having nosocomial or hospital-acquired infection[2]. The prevalence of community-acquired infection in the ICUs surveyed was 21% but the rate in other clinical areas, i.e. infectious diseases, dermatology, paediatrics, respiratory and acute medicine, was higher. In contrast, the prevalence of nosocomial infection in ICUs, at 43%, was over twice that of any other specialty[2], indicating the considerable importance of hospital-acquired infection in intensive care patients.

Data from a recent prevalence survey of European ICUs, which excluded coronary care, paediatric and special care infants units, revealed a prevalence of hospital-acquired and unit-acquired infection of 10% and 21%, respectively[3].

The high rate of ICU-acquired infection is not surprising because of the severity of patients' underlying illnesses in the ICU and the number and range of therapeutic and diagnostic procedures carried out there. Significant risk factors for infection are pulmonary artery catheterization, central venous access, stress ulcer prophylaxis, urinary catheterization, mechanical ventilation, trauma on admission and length of stay[3, 4]. A particular feature of ICUs is the range and number of intravascular devices required for effective patient management, but these predispose to line infection and bacteraemia (see Chapter 8). The incidence of infection is also related to the severity of the patient's illness on admission, as assessed by such indices as the simplified acute physiology score[5]. The importance of length of stay in predicting the development of infection in the ICU is borne out by clinical experience; the longer patients remain in the ICU, the more likely they are to acquire one or more infections. Finally, the occurrence of infection is closely correlated with poor outcome; of patients admitted to the ICU for 48 hours or more, nosocomial pneumonia was diagnosed in 17% and both nosocomial pneumonia and nosocomial bacteraemia were associated with mortality[6].

TYPES OF INFECTION

Urinary tract infection is the most prevalent nosocomial infection diagnosed in hospital patients, while lower respiratory tract infection or pneumonia is the most common community-acquired infection[2], but in the ICU urinary tract infection is relatively less common than in other clinical areas. Computerized surveillance of nosocomial infection in one UK ICU showed that the respiratory tract was the commonest site of infection (49%) followed by surgical wounds (22%) and bloodstream (17%), with the urinary tract accounting for only 12% of infections[7]. In the European prevalence study, pneumonia and lower respiratory tract infection were likewise the commonest ICU-acquired infections diagnosed (see Table 2.1)[3]. The relative frequency of different infections will of course vary according to the diagnostic criteria used (clinical, microbiological

Table 2.1 Frequency of common unit-acquired infections in the ICU.

Infection	Percentage[a]
Pneumonia	47
Lower respiratory tract	18
Urinary tract	17
Bacteraemia (laboratory confirmed)	12
Wound	7
Ear, nose and throat	5
Skin and soft tissue	5

[a] Some patients had more than one infection; adapted from reference 3.

and other), type of ICU (i.e. whether general/surgical or specialized such as cardiothoracic), the proportion of patients requiring intubation and ventilation, and the severity of the patient's illness. The criteria used to diagnose lower respiratory tract infection are especially important and therefore bronchoscopic or equivalent techniques are recommended (see Chapter 7). Also, bloodstream infection caused by coagulase-negative staphylococci such as *Staphylococcus epidermidis* may be overdiagnosed unless specimen or laboratory contamination is specifically excluded (see Chapters 4 and 8). Further details on the epidemiology of specific infections may be found in the relevant chapters. Surveillance data from medical ICUs in the USA have shown that primary bloodstream infections, pneumonia and urinary tract infections associated with invasive devices make up the great majority of nosocomial infections. Coagulase-negative staphylococcal bloodstream infection or bacteraemia was increasingly detected but enterococci were isolated more frequently than *Staphylococcus aureus*. Fungal urinary tract infections are increasing but are often asymptomatic[8].

The frequency and range of common community-acquired infections in patients admitted to the ICU also vary and include pneumonia (caused by, for example, *Streptococcus pneumoniae, Haemophilus influenzae*), surgical peritonitis (often involving anaerobic bacteria) and central nervous system (CNS) infections such as meningitis (e.g. meningococcal and pneumococcal) and encephalitis (e.g. herpes). However, a greater proportion of community-acquired pathogens are sensitive to first-line antimicrobial agents and therefore, unlike with many nosocomial pathogens, spread to other patients is less serious.

There is increasing recognition of clinical syndromes that resemble infection (probably caused by infectious agents in many instances), but where laboratory confirmation is absent. The sepsis syndrome, i.e. altered organ perfusion arising from the systemic response to infection, and the systemic inflammatory response syndrome (SIRS) are now common terms used in the ICU (see Chapter 1). These concepts may facilitate the classification of ICU patients for predicting outcome. In general, ICU patients with the sepsis syndrome are older, more likely to be admitted to the ICU as an emergency and are likely to remain in the ICU longer than patients without the sepsis syndrome, and bloodstream infection is documented in a minority of patients, i.e. in approximately 25–30%[9].

IMPORTANT ICU PATHOGENS

Bacterial pathogens predominate in the ICU but fungal infection is increasing in importance (Table 2.2). Viral infections, such as influenza during the winter months, are generally community acquired, but systemic cytomegalovirus infection is important in particular groups of patients such as the immuno-suppressed (see Chapter 12). Overall, however, viral illness is not generally very common but this may be due partly to underdiagnosis.

Gram-negative bacilli such as the Enterobacteriaceae (i.e. *Escherichia coli, Klebsiella aerogenes, Serratia marcescens*, etc.) and *P. aeruginosa* account for

Table 2.2 The major pathogens of importance in the ICU.

Pathogen	Comments
S. aureus	Methicillin resistance an increasing problem in many ICUs
Coagulase-negative staphylococci	Associated with prosthetic materials such as intravascular lines
Enterococci	Emerging pathogens; vancomycin resistance a source of some anxiety
Enterobacteriaceae (e.g. *E. coli*, *E. cloacae*)	Found in the gastrointestinal tract; outbreaks with resistant strains occur
P. aeruginosa	Survives in moist environments; intrinsically resistant to many antibiotics
Acinetobacter spp.	Emerging pathogen; outbreaks occur; effective treatment is difficult
Candida spp.	*C. albicans* and other species cause bloodstream and deep-seated infection
Anaerobes	Isolated as part of polymicrobial infection such as peritonitis or gangrene

the majority of ICU-acquired infections but Gram-positive bacteria such as *S. aureus*, coagulase-negative staphylococci (predominantly *S. epidermidis*) and the enterococci are increasing in importance. *S. aureus* was the single most commonly implicated pathogen in the recent European prevalence study, accounting for 30% of infective episodes[3]. The relative distribution of bacterial pathogens will depend on the categories of patients admitted to the ICU, e.g. patients with chronic pulmonary disease requiring ventilation in the ICU may become colonized and subsequently infected with *P. aeruginosa*, whereas in an ICU admitting many neurosurgical patients *S. epidermidis* becomes relatively more common due to cerebrospinal fluid (CSF) shunt infections. Polymicrobial (i.e. more than one pathogen) infection is a particular feature, as half of all infective episodes in the ICU are now polymicrobial[3]. Particular features of some ICU pathogens are outlined below. Antibiotic resistance among Gram-negative bacilli is of some concern but this varies from country to country and emphasizes the need for more effective preventive strategies[10].

P. aeruginosa

This waterborne bacterium is a frequent cause of lower respiratory tract infection in ventilated patients, accounting for approximately 28% of cases[3]. Whilst cross-infection does occur, the source of many infections may be endogenous with broad-spectrum antibacterial agents, many of which are relatively inactive against *P. aeruginosa*, exerting a selective pressure. Approximately half of ICU isolates are now gentamicin resistant and 25–40% are resistant to anti-pseudomonal penicillins (i.e. the ureidopenicillins), previously the mainstay of treatment[11].

Although *P. aeruginosa* may be found in the ICU environment, e.g. in sinks, its presence there is not usually clinically significant and clusters of cases or outbreaks are more likely to be due to person-to-person spread via the aerosol route or via the hands of staff. Infection with other pseudomonads such as *P. fluorescens* or *Burkholderia* (previously *Pseudomonas*) *cepacia* is less common but in the non-immunocompromised patient should prompt a search for a possible source as these bacteria survive in solutions (e.g. infusates) and moist areas.

Aerobic Gram-negative bacilli

These opportunist pathogens, which include *E. coli*, *Klebsiella* spp., *S. marcescens* and *Enterobacter cloacae*, are part of the normal large bowel flora but may emerge as pathogens during or following antibiotic use, as they are often resistant to first-line agents such as amoxycillin, commonly used in the community or in other parts of the hospital. Outbreaks caused by multiply antibiotic-resistant strains due to the production of extended β-lactamases are well described[12]. Resistance may be plasmid mediated and effective treatment of infection with these resistant strains may require a combination of an aminoglycoside (e.g. gentamicin, amikacin), if the isolate is sensitive, and a quinolone (e.g. ciprofloxacin) or a carbapenem (e.g. meropenem or imipenem/cilastin).

Acinetobacter spp.

These Gram-negative coccobacilli are emerging pathogens in the ICU because they are intrinsically resistant to many commonly used antibacterial agents. Furthermore, unlike many Gram-negative bacilli, these bacteria can survive for prolonged periods in a dry environment and this may explain the increasing occurrence of ICU outbreaks that are difficult to control. The commonest sites from which these bacteria may be recovered include the urine, the respiratory tract and wounds, but this may represent colonization only; bacteraemia and meningitis also occur, however. Emergency procedures and recent exposure to antibiotics, especially fluoroquinolones, are risk factors for acquisition but the restricted use of antibiotics significantly contributes to controlling spread[13]. Most isolates are sensitive to the carbapenems, the agents of choice in treating infection, but outbreaks caused by multi-resistant strains, including resistance to the carbapenems, have also been described[14].

Stenotrophomonas maltophilia

This bacterium, previously known as *Pseudomonas maltophilia* or *Xanthomonas maltophilia*, is increasingly recognized as a pathogen in the ICU. It is widely found in the environment and has been recovered from nosocomial sources such as dialysis machines, nebulizers, ventilation circuits and disinfectant solutions[15]. Not unlike *Acinetobacter* spp., the prevalence of this organism as a cause of lower respiratory tract infection and bacteraemia is related to previous exposure to β-lactam antibiotics, especially the carbapenems. There are relatively few effective antimicrobial agents available for therapy because of the bacterium's intrinsic resistance to many agents, but co-trimoxazole is the treatment of choice[15].

Staphylococci

S. aureus is a major pathogen in the ICU, causing lower respiratory tract infection, intravascular line sepsis, bacteraemia and wound or soft tissue infection. Methicillin-resistant *S. aureus* (MRSA) is now a significant problem in ICUs throughout Europe. Strains of MRSA are not only also resistant to all penicillin and cephalosporin antibiotics, but many are also resistant to aminoglycosides, macrolides (e.g. erythromycin) and fluoroquinolones (e.g. ciprofloxacin). Efforts undertaken to detect, treat and prevent spread represent a considerable challenge with relatively few options available for therapy[16]. MRSA strains with only intermediate susceptibility to vancomycin have been recovered from critically ill patients in the last few years, and these are causing concern as there are limited options for treatment[17].

Coagulase-negative staphylococci such as *S. epidermidis* and *S. haemolyticus* are the major cause of intravascular-associated infections and bacteraemia because of their ability to adhere to biomaterials and form 'slime' which facilitates replication and makes antibiotic treatment more difficult. Many isolates recovered from ICU patients are multiply antibiotic resistant and the mainstay of treatment is a glycopeptide antibiotic (vancomycin or teicoplanin), often in combination with an aminoglycoside or rifampicin. Vancomycin- and teicoplanin-resistant coagulase-negative staphylococci are well recognized and do occur in the ICU, causing occasional infection, and there is some anxiety that these strains may spread and become endemic.

Enterococci

Previously known as faecal streptococci, the enterococci (e.g. *Enterococcus faecalis*, *E. faecium*, *E. durans* and *E. avium*) are also an increasing problem in the ICU. Recent cephalosporin use (the cephalosporins are inactive against the enterococci and hence select for their emergence), serious underlying disease and the presence of intravascular catheters are all risk factors for colonization and infection. Should selective decontamination of the digestive tract (SDD), i.e. the topical administration of antibiotics to the buccal mucosa and via a nasogastric tube throughout the patient stay together with a parenteral third-generation cephalosporin for the first 2–4 days, become more widely used in

ICUs, enterococci may become even more prevalent as organisms colonizing and infecting patients in the ICU.

Outbreaks of vancomycin-resistant enterococci (VRE) have been described in renal units and ICUs in the UK and elsewhere, and environmental contamination with these bacteria is a significant factor. Few currently available antimicrobial agents are active against VRE. Newer compounds, currently under development, such as the glycylcyclines and oxazolidiones, show some promise[18], but the main focus currently is on good infection control practice to prevent the emergence and spread of these pathogens.

Fungi

The incidence of nosocomial fungal infection is increasing throughout the hospitals, with *Candida* spp., other yeasts and *Aspergillus* spp. being the most important pathogens. Risk factors include immunosuppression (corticosteroids, chemotherapy, malignancy), the availability of appropriate routes of infection (e.g. extensive burns, indwelling catheters) and recent exposure to antibacterial agents[19]. These risk factors are found in a high proportion of ICU patients and, not surprisingly, it is in the ICU and burn/trauma units where the greatest increase in incidence has occurred[20]. Fungal infection is often difficult to confirm with conventional laboratory methods (e.g. only about 50% of blood cultures are positive in patients with systemic candidiasis) and the isolation of either *Candida* or *Aspergillus* spp. from an ICU patient may sometimes represent colonization rather than infection, or indeed specimen contamination (e.g. *Aspergillus* isolated from sputum). Systemic *Candida* infection has increased in the ICU in recent years[4] and a greater variety of *Candida* spp. is now seen. In addition to *Candida albicans*, *C. glabrata*, *C. krusei* and *C. tropicalis* are increasingly encountered.

The significance of the different *Candida* spp. lies in their differing epidemiology and susceptibility to antifungal agents such as fluconazole, as many of the non-*albicans* species are resistant. In response to the increasing importance of *Candida* infection in ICU and surgery patients, consensus guidelines that focus on the role of the microbiology laboratory in diagnosis, management strategies, the respective roles of amphotericin B, flucytosine and fluconazole, and long-term maintenance therapy, have recently been published[21].

Key points

- Nosocomial infection is more prevalent in the ICU than in other parts of the hospital.
- Risk factors include central venous access, mechanical ventilation, stress ulcer prophylaxis with H_2 antagonists and prolonged ICU stay.
- Lower respiratory tract infection or pneumonia, urinary tract infection, bloodstream infection and wound infection are the most common ICU infections.
- *P. aeruginosa*, the Enterobacteriaceae (e.g. *E. coli*), *S. aureus* and other staphylococci are common pathogens.
- Fungi, enterococci, *Acinetobacter* spp. and *S. maltophilia* are likely to be increasingly important in the future.

REFERENCES

1. van Saene HKF, Damjanovic V, Murray AE *et al.* (1996) How to classify infections in intensive care units – the carrier state, a criterion whose time has come? *Journal of Hospital Infection* **33**: 1–12.
2. Emmerson AM, Enstone JE, Griffin M *et al.* (1996) The second national prevalence survey of infection in hospitals – overview of results. *Journal of Hospital Infection* **32**: 175–190.
3. Vincent J-L, Bihari DJ, Suter PM *et al.* (1995) The prevalence of nosocomial infection in intensive care units in Europe. Results of the European Prevalence of Infection in Intensive Care (EPIC) Study. *Journal of the American Medical Association* **274**: 639–644.
4. Jarvis WR, Edwards JR, Culver DH *et al.* (1991) Nosocomial infection rates in adults and paediatric intensive care units in the United States. *American Journal of Medicine* **91** (Suppl 3B): 185–191.
5. Girou E, Pinsard M, Auriant I *et al.* (1996) Influence of the severity of illness measured by the Simplified Acute Physiology Score (SAPS) on occurrence of nosocomial infections in ICU patients. *Journal of Hospital Infection* **34**: 131–137.
6. Fagon J-Y, Chastre J, Vuagnat A *et al.* (1996) Nosocomial pneumonia and mortality among patients in intensive care units. *Journal of the American Medical Association* **275**: 866–869.
7. Spencer RC (1994) Epidemiology of infection in ICUs. *Intensive Care Medicine* **20** (Suppl): 2–6.
8. Richards MJ, Edwards JR, Culver DH *et al.* (1999) Nosocomial infections in medical intensive care units in the United States. *Critical Care Medicine* **27**: 887–892.
9. Sands KE, Bates DW, Lanken PN *et al.* (1997) Epidemiology of sepsis syndrome in eight academic medical centers. *Journal of the American Medical Association* **278**: 234–240.
10. Hanberger H, Garcia-Rodriguez J-A, Gobernado M *et al.* (1999) Antibiotic susceptibility among aerobic Gram-negative bacilli in intensive care units in five European countries. *Journal of the American Medical Association* **281**: 67–71.

11. Spencer RC (1996) Predominant pathogens found in the European Prevalence of Infection in Intensive Care Study. *European Journal of Microbiology and Infectious Diseases* **15**: 281–285.
12. Meyer KS, Urban C, Eagan JA *et al.* (1993) Nosocomial outbreak of *Klebsiella* infection resistant to late-generation cephalosporins. *Annals of Internal Medicine* **119**: 353–358.
13. Villers D, Espaze E, Coste-Burel M *et al.* (1998) Nosocomial *Acinetobacter baumannii* infections: microbiological and clinical epidemiology. *Annals of Internal Medicine* **129**: 182–189.
14. Go ES, Urban C, Burns J *et al.* (1994) Clinical and molecular epidemiology of *Acinetobacter* infections sensitive only to polymyxin B and sulbactam. *Lancet* **344**: 1329–1332.
15. Denton M, Kerr KG (1998) Microbiological and clinical aspects of infection associated with *Stenotrophomonas maltophilia*. *Clinical Microbiology Reviews* **11**: 57–80.
16. Fraise AP (1998) Guidelines for the control of methicillin-resistant *Staphylococcus aureus*. *Journal of Antimicrobial Chemotherapy* **42**: 287–289.
17. Waldovgel FA (1999) New resistance in *Staphylococcus aureus*. *New England Journal of Medicine* **340**: 556–557.
18. Fraise AP (1996) The treatment and control of vancomycin resistant enterococci. *Journal of Antimicrobial Chemotherapy* **38**: 753–756.
19. Fridkin SK, Jarvis WR (1996) Epidemiology of nosocomial infections. *Clinical Microbiology Reviews* **9**: 499–511.
20. Flanagan PG, Barnes RA (1998) Fungal infection in the intensive care unit. *Journal of Hospital Infection* **38**: 163–177.
21. Vincent J-L, Anaissie E, Bruining H *et al.* (1998) Epidemiology, diagnosis and treatment of systemic *Candida* infection in surgical patients under intensive care. *Intensive Care Medicine* **24**: 206–216.

3 Control of infection

GENERAL CONTROL MEASURES

Many of the strategies to prevent and control the spread of infection in the intensive care unit (ICU) are part of good professional practice, e.g. hand washing before and after examining each patient, and these also contribute to high standards of patient care. Infection control measures also protect health care workers (HCWs) including ICU nurses from occupationally acquired infection. High standards of patient care contribute to hospital infection control and poor standards may be reflected by an increase in the numbers of patients acquiring nosocomial infection.

Good design and layout, with adequate staffing, are especially important in ICUs that contain patients vulnerable to infection[1]. Whilst spacious and appropriate physical facilities are clearly important, these are no substitute for well-trained and highly motivated staff, and inadequate numbers of staff contribute to the acquisition and spread of nosocomial infection. Specific issues that should be addressed when planning or upgrading an ICU include ensuring there is adequate space to minimize patient-to-patient spread of pathogens, sufficient wash handbasins, and the provision of adequate isolation facilities (Table 3.1). The need for isolation cubicles may increase in the future due to the admission of severely ill infected patients, e.g. burns patients, due to the emergence of multiply antibiotic-resistant bacteria, and due to the greater numbers of immunocompromised patients (e.g. with HIV) needing admission to the ICU and requiring protective isolation, ideally with positive-pressure air

Table 3.1   Important design features in controlling infection in the ICU.

Adequate space per patient, i.e. at least 20 m^2 per patient
Adequate hand washing and drying facilities, e.g. one handbasin for every other patient
A minimum of one isolation cubicle per six patients with facilities for negative (pressures lower than surrounding clinical areas) and positive air pressure (pressures higher than surrounding clinical areas) ventilation
Facilities for the wearing of staff protective clothing
Restricted access from the rest of the hospital
Ready access to the operating theatre and the hospital sterile services supply department

ventilation (air pressures greater in the isolation cubicle compared with surrounding clinical areas). Whilst it is important in the ICU to be able to monitor patients adequately (often by means of a central facility), at least two isolation cubicles[1] and the facility to segregate infectious from non-infectious patients are especially important during an outbreak. Not only are these necessary in effectively controlling infection, they also ensure good working conditions for HCWs in ICUs and contribute to good staff morale, which is important in promoting good professional practice. Many ICUs, however, are located in old buildings that were never designed for the needs of very ill patients and this often hampers routine infection control measures.

Hand washing and hand disinfection remain the most important measures in the prevention of cross-infection in hospital. Personnel in ICUs should wash or disinfect their hands more frequently than those in other units, such as before and after contact with each patient[2]. Hand washing removes transient flora, including important opportunist ICU pathogens (e.g. *Staphylococcus aureus* and enterococci) as well as fastidious organisms (e.g. viruses). Contaminating micro-organisms survive long enough on hands (i.e. from 30 minutes to several hours) to be transmitted to other patients. Whilst compliance with hand-washing regimens amongst HCWs including those in ICUs is often poor, it is well documented that efforts to improve hand washing result in a fall in nosocomial infection[3]. Repeated studies have shown that compliance with hand-washing regimens by medical staff is inferior to that of nurses. The use of gloves for a variety of procedures such as suctioning airways does not obviate the need for good hand-washing technique, because during removal of gloves contamination of hands may occur. Gloves should be changed between patients, otherwise organisms contaminating the outside of the glove may spread from patient to patient. Gloves should be changed when moving from 'dirty' to 'clean' activities on the same patient and, as always, hands should be washed after the removal of gloves. Bed linen from patients in isolation should be placed in an alginate bag, which is then placed in a second bag for subsequent disposal[4].

Good hand-washing technique involves adequate washing, rinsing and drying of the front and backs of the hands including the web spaces, using elbow-operated water taps and a liquid disinfectant soap dispenser, followed by drying with paper towels disposed of in a foot-operated bin (Plate 1). Where there are insufficient wash handbasins, the provision of alcoholic handrubs at each bed may encourage hand washing between patients. Good practice such as the use of an aseptic technique and appropriate hand washing before the insertion of a central line is also important in minimizing the risk of unit-acquired infection. Appropriate decontamination by disinfection or sterilization of instruments and equipment is often taken for granted in the ICU. Sterilization, i.e. the removal of all microbes including bacterial spores, is required for equipment used in sterile body tissues whereas disinfection, i.e. the removal of adequate numbers of potentially pathogenic microbes to make an instrument safe, may be sufficient for equipment used in contact with the skin and mucous membranes[5]. Cleaning, i.e. washing with detergent, is essential before either of the above as this dramatically reduces the bioburden. However, increasingly there are

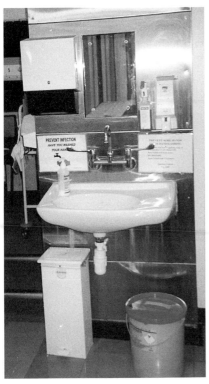

Plate 1 Hand-washing facilities including elbow-operated taps, soap/disinfectant dispenser, paper towels and foot-operated bin.

difficulties faced by the use of heat-sensitive equipment in sterile sites which are difficult to decontaminate adequately using conventional methodologies. Ethylene oxide as a sterilant is not always available locally but newer technologies such as the use of hydrogen peroxide, gas plasma and chlorine dioxide show some promise[5]. In addition to the requirement to reduce the bioburden on instruments and equipment, environmental cleanliness is also important. ICUs and all other clinical areas should be cleaned regularly to minimize the potential for opportunist pathogens to survive in the inanimate environment and subsequently spread to patients.

Close liaison between ICU staff and infection control personnel will heighten awareness of infection, help maintain high professional standards and contribute to clinical audit. In particular, ICU staff should be encouraged to inform infection control staff of outbreaks early on, discuss relevant aspects of any new procedure introduced or equipment purchased, and establish joint initiatives in the surveillance of infection and clinical audit. Issues contributing to patient care include monitoring the incidence of central intravenous catheter infections, ensuring compliance with guidelines for the control of methicillin-resistant *S. aureus* (MRSA) in hospitals[6], which increasingly focus on high-risk areas such as ICUs, and the decontamination of bronchoscopes, which should include cleaning with detergent, contact with a disinfectant for a specified period, and rinsing in sterile water to minimize contamination with atypical mycobacteria[7].

Measures important for the control of MRSA infections include screening at-risk patients on admission, isolating or cohorting positive patients, measures to reduce colonization such as the use of topical mupirocin, the use of gloves and disposable aprons and, of course, hand washing.

OCCUPATIONAL HEALTH

Close liaison between the ICU, the infection control team and the hospital occupational health department (OHD) is also important in preventing infection in ICU patients and staff by screening, immunization and education. Airborne infections occupationally acquired by HCWs such as tuberculosis, influenza and varicella are preventable by standard infection control measures and the appropriate vaccination of staff[8]. Staff working in the ICU are at least as vulnerable as other HCWs because high-risk patients may be admitted to the ICU (e.g. open tuberculosis) and their care requires greater staff–patient contact. Chickenpox (varicella) frequently causes concern amongst staff, especially pregnant staff. Susceptible staff, i.e. those who are not immune and who have been exposed to varicella, should not attend 'at-risk' immunocompromised, obstetric or neonatal patients for 7–21 days after contact; if this is not possible, they should be given leave of absence[9]. A previous history of chickenpox is, however, a reliable indicator of immunity but in staff who are uncertain whether they have had varicella infection previously it may be worthwhile assessing immune status on commencing work in the ICU. Other potential occupationally acquired infections in the ICU that are of increasing concern are blood-borne pathogens such as HIV, hepatitis B virus (HBV) and hepatitis C virus (HCV) and pathogens acquired through the faecal–oral route such as *Salmonella* and hepatitis A virus. Various guidelines and recommendations have been issued by governmental and professional bodies to minimize the risk of blood-borne infections. These emphasize good professional practice (e.g. wearing gloves), the safe disposal of needles, vaccination against hepatitis B and early self-referral for suspected or confirmed HIV infection[10]. The safe and efficient disposal of medical waste continues to pose challenges but is essential to protect HCWs and the public, and address wider environmental issues.

The immunization requirements of ICU staff and other HCWs will vary according to the country, the efficacy of vaccines available and the patient population admitted to the ICU. ICU staff should be protected against hepatitis B, and preferably against measles, mumps and rubella either through natural infection or following a course of vaccination, and there may also be a place for immunization against hepatitis A and varicella-zoster[11]. Although there has been a reassessment of the efficacy and use of BCG as a public health measure to prevent tuberculosis, it seems prudent to continue to recommend it for HCWs in countries where this disease is prevalent, even more so following the emergence of multi-drug-resistant strains. In North America, the use of BCG is not widespread because of the low incidence of tuberculosis in the population and because vaccination complicates the diagnosis of tuberculosis by skin testing.

ANTIBIOTIC USE

Whilst the availability of effective antimicrobial agents represents one of the great medical advances of the last 60 years, there is increasing awareness that antibiotics are a precious resource whose use should be controlled to prevent the emergence of resistance, to contain health care costs and to ensure that current agents continue to remain useful. A recent major report on anti-microbial resistance in the UK has recommended the development and use of computer-aided decision-support systems for improving the prescribing of antimicrobial agents in hospitals[12]. Even in ICUs where the value of antibiotics is probably better appreciated than in many other clinical areas, there is much room for improvement. Strategic goals for optimizing antibiotic use and for detecting and reporting the emergence of antibiotic resistance in hospitals are available[13]. All these issues are therefore important in the ICU, where the prevalence of antibiotic resistance is likely to be greater and where the consequences of infection with resistant bacteria are even more serious. Education of all prescribers, both in hospitals and in the community, in the sensible use of antibiotics is important and this must include feedback on patterns of antibiotic use and information on the emergence and transmission of resistant strains.

The principles of good antimicrobial practice in the ICU are similar to those in the rest of the hospital and are best set out in an antibiotic policy. In the UK, 95% of hospitals have policies on antibiotic treatment and antibiotic prophylaxis and 52% of hospitals have educational campaigns[14]. The complexity of infections in the ICU often justifies a specific unit policy as the incidence of infection is high, resistance is more likely to emerge as ICU patients often require more than one course of antibiotics, and the choice of agent and dosage will be influenced by factors such as multi-organ failure. There is, however, no substitute for frequent if not daily visits to the ICU by medical microbiologists or infectious disease physicians. Key principles in the use of antimicrobial agents for prophylaxis and treatment are outlined in Table 3.2. The prescribing of antibiotics for prophylaxis often takes place before admission to the ICU but close liaison between other clinicians, anaesthetists, intensivists and micro-biologists can lead to significant improvements, especially if ICU policies are based on general principles[15]. Monitoring the use of prophylactic antibiotics can be assessed with reference to quality standards produced following multi-disciplinary consensus[16]. The cycling of antibiotics (i.e. varying the agents used in an ordered way over time) in specialized units such as ICUs, together with strict control over the use of certain agents, has been advocated to prevent the emergence of resistance when fewer new antibacterial agents are being developed[17]. This may not be feasible in some ICUs, however, where there may already be few options for treatment because of widespread antibiotic resistance.

Selective decontamination of the digestive tract (SDD) is used in some ICUs as part of a strategy to reduce unit-acquired infection. This consists of topical antimicrobial agents applied to the oral mucosa and via a nasogastric tube (often accompanied by an intravenous extended-spectrum cephalosporin

Table 3.2 Principles of good antibiotic use in the ICU.

Therapeutic use

Take specimens before starting or changing antibiotics and be guided by the
  results

Use narrow-spectrum (e.g. benzyl penicillin) rather than broad-spectrum (e.g.
  cefotaxime) antibiotics where the pathogen is known and susceptible

Reserve new or expensive agents for second- or even third-line treatment

Avoid multiple agents unless treating difficult or polymicrobial infection

Keep antibiotic courses short, i.e. 5–7 days; review antibiotics daily

---

Surgical prophylaxis

Administer the first dose at induction of anaesthesia, before a tourniquet is
  inflated, to ensure maximum tissue levels; a second dose of most β-lactams
  is required if the procedure lasts >3 hours or there is major blood loss

If possible, avoid using the same agent(s) for prophylaxis and treatment

Two or three doses at most are sufficient; subsequent doses are *not* prophylaxis!

---

administered for the first 3–4 days of ICU stay) to prevent colonization with opportunist pathogens such as coliforms and to preserve the protective effect of the predominantly anaerobic flora of the gastrointestinal tract. Many trials and meta-analyses have confirmed that, whilst SDD reduces the incidence of colonization and infection with potential pathogens, there is only a modest effect on mortality and the duration of ICU stay in most studies. Despite the potential benefits in some patients, the routine use of SDD remains somewhat controversial[18, 19] but may have a place in certain patients, such as those who have experienced multiple trauma[20]. However, if the most effective form of prophylaxis (i.e. topical and intravenous agents) is used, it is suggested that the incidence of respiratory tract infection may be reduced by 65% and the total mortality rate reduced by 20%[19]. Despite this, continuing concerns over the emergence of multiply resistant bacteria and the relatively high cost of most SDD regimens have inhibited many ICUs from adopting this approach.

ORGANISM-RELATED ISSUES

Conventional pathogens

β-Haemolytic streptococcus group A (BHSA), also known as S. *pyogenes*, is a virulent and infectious pathogen that causes severe systemic infection, with or without bacteraemia, and necrotizing cellulitis. Patients with BHSA should be isolated in a single cubicle, preferably with negative air pressure ventilation, and gowns and aprons should be used by staff during patient contact. Infectivity is significantly reduced after 48–72 hours of antimicrobial therapy.

Tuberculosis continues to remain important and a high index of suspicion is needed when caring for patients in at-risk groups such as immigrants, alcoholics or HIV-positive patients. Notification to public health authorities to facilitate follow-up of relatives and others, isolation of all smear-positive cases and identification of patient and staff contacts are important in minimizing spread. Routine periodic chest radiography is not necessary for HCWs who have been vaccinated with BCG as it is very uncommon for hospital staff to acquire tuberculosis from patients[21].

Diphtheria should be considered in the differential diagnosis of any patient admitted to the ICU with severe tonsillitis compromising the integrity of the airway and requiring intubation, if there is no history of vaccination, and especially in any patient who has worked or travelled extensively in areas where vaccination rates are low (see Chapter 7).

In sending a specimen for microbiological confirmation, culture for *Corynebacterium diphtheriae* should be requested as this is no longer routine in many microbiology laboratories and the medical microbiologist should be notified. Spread of *C. diphtheriae* is by the airborne route and culture-positive or clinically suspected patients should be isolated in a cubicle with negative air pressure ventilation. Further details on measures to control the spread of specific pathogens may be found elsewhere[4].

Multi-resistant bacteria

Antibiotic-resistant bacteria are more common in the ICU because of the many debilitated, vulnerable patients found there who often require repeated courses of antibiotics and whose care necessitates considerable handling by nursing and other staff. Problem bacteria include MRSA, vancomycin-resistant enterococci (VRE) for which there are few treatment options available[22], as well as multi-resistant Gram-negative bacilli. Patient isolation or cohorting (i.e. segregating positive patients from negative patients with designated staff), hand washing, environmental cleaning and selective screening of patient contacts and staff are recommended for the control of MRSA and VRE[6, 23]. The emergence of MRSA strains with reduced susceptibility to vancomycin is of particular concern in ICUs but similar measures including prudent antibiotic use and patient isolation are recommended to prevent spread[24]. Similar measures are adopted for controlling resistant Gram-negative bacilli and should be carried out following the advice of the hospital infection control team.

Acinetobacter spp., small Gram-negative coccobacilli, are emerging pathogens in many ICUs. Only 36% of units recently surveyed in Great Britain and Ireland had not isolated these Gram-negative bacteria during the previous 12 months but outbreaks caused by these bacteria had occurred in 16%[25]. This development may reflect the changing demography of ICU patients, the capacity of these bacteria to persist in the ICU environment and, finally, the frequent and all too prevalent inappropriate use of antibiotics.

Blood-borne viruses

Inoculation risk incidents, e.g. needle stick injuries, are relatively common in the ICU, and the risk of occupationally acquired HIV, HBV and HCV is a genuine concern. First-aid measures following such incidents, e.g. encouraging the wound to bleed and washing in running water, should be instituted and a risk assessment made of the likelihood of subsequent infection. All such incidences should also be reported to senior staff and the OHD. Immunization against HBV and good practice, including the safe disposal of sharps, covering broken skin when carrying out a procedure, and the use of gloves when contamination with blood is likely during a procedure, will minimize the risk. Incidents in which the acquisition of one or more of these viruses is possible should be fully documented to facilitate a general assessment of the likely risk of infection[8, 26]. Decisions on whether or not a booster dose of HBV vaccine or the administration of hepatitis B immunoglobulin is required can then be made in consultation with the OHD and the infection control team, and in accordance with relevant policies. Post-exposure prophylaxis with anti-retroviral agents is recommended after a careful assessment of the nature of the injury and the source of the sharp or needle has been carried out in order to minimize the risk of occupationally acquired HIV infection[27].

As in all aspects of infection control and occupational health, the key is prevention. This includes the use of universal precautions (e.g. wearing gloves when handling body fluids irrespective of source), the safe disposal of sharps in appropriate sharps boxes and the appropriate management of blood spillages with disinfectants according to local policies. Protective clothing is required when there is likely to be contact with fluids and hence gowns or plastic aprons should be used in these circumstances. Masks and eye protection (i.e. goggles or eye visors) should be worn if there is likely to be splashing with blood[4].

Key points

- Strategies to control infection are part of good professional practice, enhance the overall quality of patient care and protect health care workers from occupational infection.
- Hand washing, adequate space and the provision of isolation cubicles are all important measures in minimizing unit-acquired infection.
- The sensible and rational use of antibiotics for treatment and prophylaxis minimizes the emergence of multiply antibiotic-resistant bacteria.
- SDD is not recommended as a routine measure to prevent or control ICU infection in all patients.
- Close liaison between the ICU, occupational health department and the infection control team is important in preventing occupationally acquired infections such as hepatitis.

REFERENCES

1. Intensive Care Society (1997) *Standards for Intensive Care Units*. ICS, London.
2. Daschner FD (1985) Useful and useless hygienic techniques in intensive care units. *Intensive Care Medicine* **11**: 280–283.
3. Nyström B (1994) Impact of hand washing on mortality in intensive care; examination of the evidence. *Infection Control and Hospital Epidemiology* **15**: 435–436.
4. Philpott-Howard J, Casewell M (1994) *Hospital Infection Control. Policies and Practical Procedures*. WB Saunders, London.
5. Rutala WA, Weber DJ (1996) Low-temperature sterilization technologies: do we need to redefine 'sterilization'? *Infection Control and Hospital Epidemiology* **17**: 87–91.
6. Combined Working Party of the Hospital Infection Society, the British Society for Antimicrobial Chemotherapy and the Infection Control Nurses Association (1998) Working party report. Revised guidelines for the control of methicillin-resistant *Staphylococcus aureus* infection in hospitals. *Journal of Hospital Infection* **39**: 253–290.
7. Uttley AHC, Simpson RA (1994) Audit of bronchoscope disinfection; a survey of procedures in England and Wales and incidents of mycobacterial contamination. *Journal of Hospital Infection* **26**: 301–308.
8. Sepkowitz KA (1996) Occupationally acquired infections in health care workers. Part I. *Annals of Internal Medicine* **125**: 826–834.
9. Burns SM, Mitchell-Heggs N, Carrington D (1998) Occupational and infection control aspects of varicella. *Journal of Infection* **36** (Suppl 1): 73–78.
10. Association of Anaesthetists of Great Britain and Ireland (1992) *HIV and Other Blood-borne Viruses – Guidance for Anaesthetists*. AAGBI, London.
11. Sepkowitz KA (1996) Occupationally acquired infections in health care workers. Part II. *Annals of Internal Medicine* **125**: 917–928.
12. Standing Medical Advisory Committee Subgroup on Antimicrobial Resistance (1998) *The Path of Least Resistance*. Department of Health, London.
13. Goldmann DA, Weinstein RA, Wenzel RP et al. (1996) Strategies to prevent and control the emergence and spread of antimicrobial-resistant microorganisms in hospitals: a challenge to hospital leadership. *Journal of the American Medical Association* **275**: 234–240.
14. Working Party of the British Society for Antimicrobial Chemotherapy (1994) Hospital antibiotic control measures in the UK. *Journal of Antimicrobial Chemotherapy* **34**: 21–42.
15. Timms J, Humphreys H (1997) Antimicrobial prophylaxis in the intensive care unit. *Current Anaesthesia and Critical Care* **8**: 133–138.
16. Dellinger EP, Gross PA, Barrett TL et al. (1994) Quality standard for antimicrobial prophylaxis in surgical procedures. *Clinical Infectious Diseases* **18**: 422–427.
17. Sanders WE, Sanders CC (1996) Cycling of antibiotics: an approach to circumvent resistance in specialized units of the hospital. *Clinical Microbiology and Infection* **1**: 223–225.
18. Bonten MJM, Weinstein RA (1996) Selective decontamination of the digestive tract: a measure whose time has passed? *Current Opinion in Infectious Diseases* **9**: 270–275.
19. D'Amico R, Pifferi S, Leonetti C et al. (1998) Effectiveness of antibiotic prophylaxis in critically ill adult patients: systematic review of randomized controlled trials. *British Medical Journal* **316**: 1275–1285.

20. Humphreys H (1994) The future role of selective decontamination of the digestive tract (SDD) in trauma. *Care of the Critically Ill* **10**: 170–172.
21. Joint Tuberculosis Committee of the British Thoracic Society (1994) Control and prevention of tuberculosis in the United Kingdom: Code of Practice 1994. *Thorax* **49**: 1193–1200.
22. Michel M, Gutmann L (1997) Methicillin-resistant *Staphylococcus aureus* and vancomycin-resistant enterococci: therapeutic realities and possibilities. *Lancet* **349**: 1901–1906.
23. Chadwick PR, Chadwick CD, Oppenheim BA (1996) Report of a meeting on the epidemiology and control of glycopeptide-resistant enterococci. *Journal of Hospital Infection* **33**: 83–92.
24. Smith TL, Pearson ML, Wilcox KR et al. (1999) Emergence of vancomycin resistance in *Staphylococcus aureus*. *New England Journal of Medicine* **340**: 493–501.
25. Humphreys H, Towner KJ (1997) Impact of *Acinetobacter* spp. in intensive care units in Great Britain and Ireland. *Journal of Hospital Infection* **37**: 281–286.
26. Gerberding JL (1995) Management of occupational exposures to blood-borne viruses. *New England Journal of Medicine* **322**: 444–451.
27. Department of Health (1997) *Guidelines on post-exposure prophylaxis for health care workers occupationally exposed to HIV*. Department of Health, London.

4 Diagnosis of infection

Clinical assessment remains the first step in diagnosing infection and in guiding appropriate treatment. Frequent auscultation of the heart and lungs and simple inspection of possible sites of infection such as the sacral area for pressure sores, the removal of dressings to exclude wound or intravascular line-site infection and fundoscopy in patients at risk for systemic *Candida* infection are essential, and will help determine which laboratory or radiological investigations should be undertaken. Each intensive care unit (ICU) should establish its own policies for evaluating fever as an indicator of infection that take account of the type of ICU (i.e. general, neurosurgery), the patient population, the relative numbers of immunosuppressed or immunocompetent patients and the recent occurrence of epidemics (e.g. methicillin-resistant *Staphylococcus aureus*; MRSA)[1]. Figure 4.1 outlines the general principles of the management of ICU patients with suspected infection. However, there are many situations even in critically ill patients where it may be appropriate to hold off administering antibiotics if the patient is clinically stable whilst awaiting the results of investigations. The unnecessary or excessive use of antibiotics is a major factor in the emergence of resistance.

NON-MICROBIOLOGICAL INVESTIGATIONS

Microbiological investigations determine the cause of infection and guide therapy, but other tests may provide the first clue to the presence of infection (e.g. consolidation on chest X-ray, raised peripheral white cell count), or may occasionally indicate the aetiology (e.g. cold agglutinins suggesting infection with *Mycoplasma pneumoniae*).

Laboratory tests

A raised peripheral white cell count and differential may sometimes be useful as an indicator of possible infection, but a low count due to marrow suppression may occur in severe systemic infection. Non-infective conditions such as the acute respiratory distress syndrome are sometimes accompanied by a raised white cell count and many patients with infection have a normal cell count. Consequently, the results of the white cell count and differential should always be interpreted with caution. The same can be said of the erythrocyte sedimentation rate (ESR) and C-reactive protein (CRP), an acute-phase protein, and relatively crude indicators of infection. Whilst a raised CRP level of 200–300 mg l^{-1}

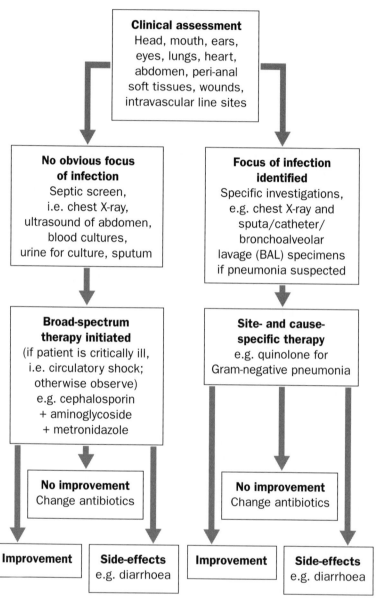

Figure 4.1 Approach to the management of infection.

(normal 6–10 mg l^{-1}) may be more indicative of bacterial infection, previous reports suggesting a role in the monitoring of infection in adult and paediatric neutropenic patients have not been confirmed.

The physiological changes that arise during sepsis have also been proposed as markers of infection; in patients with circulatory shock due to infection, blood lactate levels are raised and declining levels subsequently are associated with the successful resuscitation of septic shock[2]. Monitoring cytokine levels to predict bacteraemia or to indicate when antimicrobial therapy is indicated have been studied recently; interleukin 6 (IL-6) and tumour necrosis factor (TNF) are better markers of bacteraemia than CRP[3]. However, there is considerable over-lap in plasma levels between bacteraemic and non-bacteraemic patients and this approach still requires validation in multiple centres.

Radiological and imaging investigations

Radiography, ultrasonography (US), computed tomography (CT), nuclear and magnetic resonance imaging (MRI) are important in diagnosing infection, but CT and MRI are not always available and require the patient to be transferred temporarily out of the ICU. Plain X-rays of the chest and abdomen, and X-rays of the skull, sinuses and long bones when indicated, are the initial imaging investigations of choice. Positive findings may preclude the necessity for more complicated and expensive investigations.

After plain X-rays, US is the investigation of choice for many ICU patients as it allows non-invasive evaluation of major abdominal organ pathology as well as diagnostic aspirations, and drainage. For example, US has a sensitivity of 95% for detecting gallstones[4], it is the investigation of choice for detecting biliary sludge and hepatic abscesses >2 cm, and it has had a major impact on the diagnosis of hepatic candidiasis in patients following anti-cancer chemotherapy or bone marrow transplantation[4]. Drainage of pyogenic abscesses may be undertaken if there is a defined abscess of sufficient size, a safe route for drainage and acceptable clotting indices. However, the presence of drains, dressings, stomas, sinuses or skin changes may greatly affect the usefulness of US as all these impair impedance flow (Figure 4.2).

Unlike US, the need to transport the patient to the radiology department is a major disadvantage of CT; MRI is still available only in the larger centres. CT of the abdomen is helpful in diagnosing pancreatic abscesses when gas bubbles are very suggestive of infection[5], but differentiation from pseudocysts, haematomas, etc. is very much dependent on the skill and expertise of the radiologist. CT or MRI remains the investigation of choice for intracranial infections, e.g. herpes encephalitis, and in the immunosuppressed patient to diagnose toxoplasmosis (Figure 4.3).

Scintigraphic or nuclear medicine procedures are useful in patients if US and CT or MRI scans are negative. Nuclear medicine scans involve the intravenous injection of a radiopharmaceutical followed by imaging 24–48 hours later. Nuclear medicine scans are whole-body investigations, and may detect early or diffuse infection, unlike US or CT scans, but, like these, the procedure cannot be carried out in the ICU. Another disadvantage is that the results are not available for 24–48 hours, a relatively long time in the acutely ill patient. Nonetheless, as second-line investigations, gallium citrate scans can be very helpful in the diagnosis of lung infections or in assessing pulmonary fibrotic diseases such as vasculitis, and indium-leukocyte scintigraphy has a role in the detection of abdominal and pelvic infection (Figure 4.4)[6].

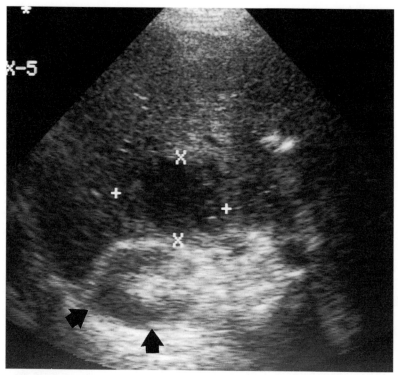

Figure 4.2 Liver abscess (delineated by 'X' and '+') anterior to the right kidney (arrows).

MICROBIOLOGICAL INVESTIGATIONS

The isolation of a pathogen and antibiotic susceptibility tests (in the case of bacteria) provide the greatest reassurance regarding the diagnosis and correct treatment of infection. However, this ideal is frequently not achieved because antimicrobial agents have often been started before appropriate investigations are carried out, or because of limitations in laboratory methods. Although there is an increasing number of laboratory techniques available, e.g. microscopy and culture, certain issues need to be considered regarding the number, type and timing of specimens (Table 4.1). Furthermore, repeated clinical assessment of the patient remains essential as this will guide which investigations are a priority.

Diagnostic laboratories have to balance the need to provide a comprehensive and accurate result with the requirement to provide a result that is timely in the acutely ill patient; bacteriology results that take more than 2 days quickly lose their relevance. Clinical details to ensure that the most appropriate tests are done in the laboratory are essential and must accompany laboratory requests. For example, it is essential that clinical features accompany bronchoscopy specimens as tests for *Legionella*, *Mycoplasma* and *Chlamydia* are not always routine. The following laboratory techniques are currently available.

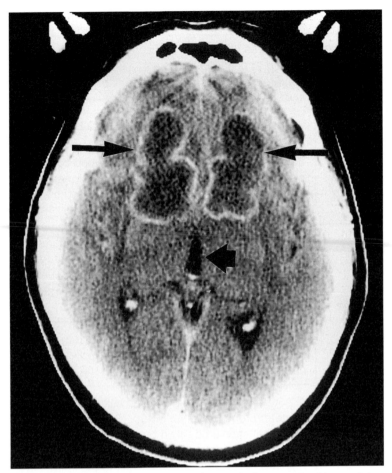

Figure 4.3 Bilateral frontal abscesses (arrows) characterized by peripheral contrast enhancement pattern with white edges.

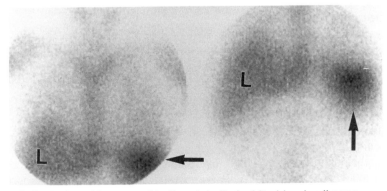

Figure 4.4 Delayed images of indium-labelled white blood cell scan demonstrating marked radiotracer uptake in spleen (arrows). Liver is indicated by 'L'.

Table 4.1 A rational approach to using the microbiology laboratory.

When?	As soon as infection is suspected and before therapy is started or changed. It is preferable if at all possible to carry out complicated investigations during normal working hours when full laboratory expertise is available
Which?	Good-quality specimens, e.g. pus > swabs, and those from normally sterile sites such as blood (blood cultures), cerebrospinal fluid (CSF), abdomen (peritoneal aspirates). Other specimens, e.g. sputa and wound swabs, are less specific
How many?	No more than two specimens (three if endocarditis is suspected) are usually required but blood cultures should be repeated if the patient remains pyrexial or unstable. Follow-up serum specimens are usually required for serological diagnosis
How often?	Daily or twice-daily clinical assessments may be required in pyrexial patients or those who are clinically unstable to determine the frequency of tests
What?	A 'sepsis screen' (e.g. two blood cultures, urine, respiratory catheter/bronchoalveolar lavage (BAL), drainage fluids, pus or swabs) should be taken but discussion with a microbiologist/infectious disease physician should occur regularly to tailor the investigations to the individual patient

Microscopy

The Gram stain, one of the simplest, cheapest and most rapid of investigations, may provide a presumptive diagnosis in a matter of minutes, e.g. in the diagnosis of pneumonia (Gram-positive diplococci – *Streptococcus pneumoniae*; see Plate 2), septic arthritis (e.g. Gram-positive cocci in clusters – *S. aureus*) or candidaemia (budding yeasts). Although specific, the Gram stain lacks sensitivity and will be diagnostic in a minority of patients. The Ziehl–Neelsen or auramine stain on a tracheal aspirate or sputum may confirm tuberculosis and fluorescent microscopy of throat washings or bronchoalveolar lavage (BAL), which combines microscopy with antigen detection (see below), may be used to confirm influenza, *Legionella* or *Pneumocystis carinii*. Electron microscopy is helpful in confirming the presence of herpes viruses in vesicles and, finally, tissue biopsies taken for histological examination, including special stains, may diagnose fungal infection.

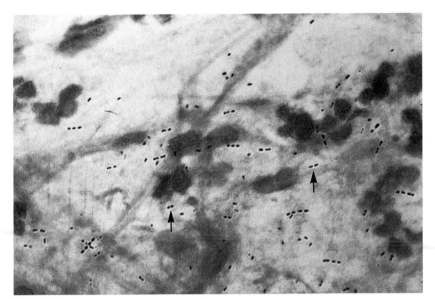

Plate 2 Gram stain of purulent sputum as indicated by the presence of 'pus' cells. Numerous Gram-positive diplococci are present (arrows).

Culture

Culture provides an isolate that can be tested for antibiotic sensitivity in the case of bacteria. Isolates can also be typed and this may assist in determining the source, and subsequent spread, of infection. Most bacteria are recovered after 24–48 hours incubation but fungi may take longer and conventional virus culture takes a week or more. Unless specific clinical details are provided with the specimen, appropriate artificial media may not be used, e.g. in neutropenic patients *Aspergillus* spp. may not be isolated from blood and chocolate agar which are routinely used (Plate 3). Culture for viruses, *Chlamydia* and *Rickettsia* requires tissue culture facilities which are usually more time consuming and are not available in every hospital. Consequently, there is increasing use of antigen detection for viruses combined with tissue culture to speed up diagnosis, e.g. the detection of early antigen fluorescent foci (DEAFF) test for cytomegalovirus (CMV), which may be positive within 48 hours.

Serology

Methods to detect antibodies to pathogens are now more efficient following the introduction of automated enzyme immunoassays (EIAs), but a serological diagnosis is not usually rapid unless the patient has been ill for some time, when the first antibody titre may be increased. For example, antibodies are unlikely to be present in the serum of a patient presenting with acute influenza unless the patient has been ill for 5–7 days or more, and therefore a repeat specimen is usually required to demonstrate a fourfold or greater rise in antibody titre. Assays to detect the presence of immunoglobulin M (IgM) (e.g.

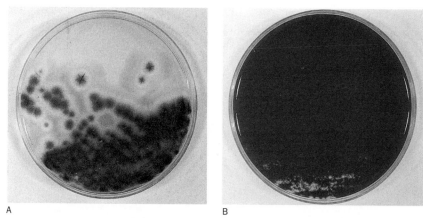

Plate 3 Heavy growth of *Aspergillus* spp. on Saboraud agar (A) compared with blood agar (B).

hepatitis A, parvovirus), indicating recent or acute infection, are useful but are not always available for a particular pathogen, or may not be technically feasible in the laboratory. In general, serum should be taken as soon as possible from ICU patients considered to be infected but in whom the aetiology is uncertain, e.g. viral pneumonia, for serological examination.

Antigen detection

Because of the delay required to culture many pathogens, antigen detection has many attractions since, in addition to being theoretically faster, it does not require viable organisms. This approach has been in use for many years in the diagnosis of hepatitis, e.g. hepatitis B surface antigen, one of the earliest markers of acute hepatitis B. Antigen detection usually requires the use in the laboratory of commercially available antibodies that will react with microbial antigens. Antibody–antigen reactions may be detected by fluorescent microscopy where fluorescent-labelled antibodies bind specific antigen, as in the microscopic detection of *Legionella* in respiratory specimens (Plate 4). There has been much interest in detecting fungal antigenaemia to diagnose systemic candidaemia as blood cultures are positive in only 40–50% of cases. However, this has not proven as successful as originally thought, since antigenaemia is intermittent and is often of very short duration. For many opportunist pathogens, detecting microbial nucleic acid using the polymerase chain reaction (PCR) has overtaken developments in antigen detection as this should theoretically be more sensitive, requiring small numbers of microbes or nucleic acid which may or may not be viable (see below).

Molecular techniques

Newer technology including gene probes, enzymes that cut DNA at specific sites and PCR will have an increasing role to play in diagnosis, epidemiological investigations to trace the spread of infection, and determining antibiotic

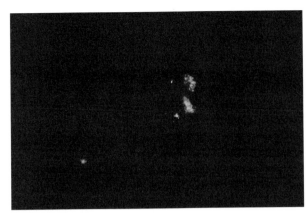

Plate 4 Diagnosis of influenza A confirmed by antigen detection in bronchoalveolar lavage specimen using specific fluorescent antibodies.

resistance[7]. In particular, PCR offers great potential in the diagnosis of infection caused by organisms that are difficult to grow (e.g. *Legionella*) or take a long time (e.g. tuberculosis).

Essentially PCR involves a series of heating and cooling phases which together with primers (complementary strands of DNA) and the enzyme DNA polymerase facilitates the production of multiple copies of DNA, hence resulting in the detection of specific DNA. Theoretically, PCR can detect a single gene sequence, but in practice a more realistic level of sensitivity is probably of the order of 100–1000 cells because many clinical specimens, especially those from normally non-sterile sites such as sputum, are more complex to assay and contain biological inhibitors that affect PCR. However, PCR can provide a result in 4–6 hours which is a significant improvement, especially compared with viral culture. A recent review indicates how PCR can be used to diagnose a wide range of respiratory infections including *S. pneumoniae*, tuberculosis and the less common causes of pneumonia[8].

However, it is in the area of the diagnosis of viral infections that PCR is having, and is likely to continue to have, an increasing impact because results from viral culture may take weeks. Even newer antigen detection systems such as DEAFF for the diagnosis of CMV (see above) are labour intensive and relatively insensitive. Commercial systems are now available for the detection of CMV nucleic acid in biological fluids and may be used early in BAL specimens to identify those patients vulnerable to developing CMV pneumonitis and who are therefore likely to benefit from the early introduction of anti-CMV agents. Similarly, the diagnosis of viral encephalitis has in the past been hampered by the inaccessibility of the infected area and delays in viral culture. Whilst CT scans and even the electroencephalogram (EEG) may be suggestive, a specific diagnosis is essential for herpes encephalitis, as treatment with aciclovir must be started as soon as possible if it is to be effective. Examination of CSF by PCR for the detection of herpes gene sequences is now part of routine laboratory investigations. The laboratory protocol should be able to distinguish herpes simplex virus (HSV) type 1 from type 2, and viral DNA is usually detectable at the onset of neurological symptoms and for 5 days after therapy has started[9]. Furthermore, although 10 days of treatment is usually effective, aciclovir should be continued for as long as the CSF is PCR positive if the clinical response is slow.

More recently, the development of multiplex PCR to detect a number of different viral genomes has been developed and evaluated. Approximately 8% of CSF specimens were positive and the relatively high incidence of HSV2 was one of the surprising findings[10]. The use of such assays to detect two or more pathogens is likely to become more common in the years ahead. Similarly, studies involving the use of a panfungal PCR assay to detect subunit ribosomal RNA gene sequences of two major fungal organism groups has recently been shown to have a sensitivity of four organisms per millilitre of blood and can detect a wide range of fungal pathogens[11]. It is likely that such an assay or something similar will be routinely available within a couple of years as blood cultures are not sensitive enough.

Diagnosis of bacterial infection due to resistant organisms is of great importance as inappropriate therapy usually leads to an unfavourable outcome and many of these organisms spread easily. The detection of MRSA currently takes 48–72 hours, as the bacterium must first be isolated and sensitivity tests then carried out. The *mecA* gene, which codes for methicillin resistance, is absent from susceptible staphylococcal isolates and this can be used to detect MRSA isolates. A multiplex PCR assay (to detect genes indicative of both *S. aureus* and methicillin resistance) was compared with culture and confirmed the presence of MRSA in culture-positive endotracheal specimens, and correctly detected MRSA in additional specimens[12].

Whilst PCR and other molecular techniques require careful validation in the clinical context, it is likely that for certain infections these will become the diagnostic approach of choice, as their enhanced sensitivity and speed outweigh the additional expense.

SPECIFIC INVESTIGATIONS FOR SOME LIFE-THREATENING INFECTIONS

The range of available laboratory and other techniques has been briefly described above but it is often difficult to choose the most appropriate tests at the right time. If in doubt, seek advice from laboratory staff or from micro-biologists and infectious disease physicians. What follows is an outline of the important initial investigations in selected life-threatening infections; more details are provided on these and other infections in the relevant chapters. Further tests may be required later depending on the clinical course, or the results of initial investigations.

Systemic sepsis

Blood cultures remain the single most important investigation in the acutely ill febrile patient, and the key points of this investigation are outlined in Table 4.2.

Table 4.2 Diagnostic approach to the patient with systemic sepsis.

Blood cultures

Clean skin first with disinfectant, e.g. povidone–iodine or alcohol, and allow to dry before venepuncture

Take 10–15 ml per blood culture set

Take two sets at a time, one through an intravascular line, if this is a suspected source

Repeat blood cultures if the patient remains pyrexial and if clinically indicated, e.g. haemodynamically unstable

Other investigations

Urine, but CSUs are often chronically colonized with potential pathogens and the urinary white cell count may be increased in the absence of infection due to the presence of a 'foreign body'

Review all intravascular lines; removed lines should be sent for culture

Fresh fluid from drainage sites should be sent for culture

Endotracheal aspirates/sputa or preferably BAL/PBS (see below) if lower respiratory infection suspected

Imaging (e.g. US) and surgical exploration and drainage should be considered

Blood films for malaria if patient has returned from or travelled through an endemic area

CSU, catheter specimen of urine; BAL, bronchoalveolar lavage; PBS, protected brush or catheter specimen; US, ultrasonography.

Except when infective endocarditis is suspected (see Chapter 13), no more than two blood culture sets (i.e. four bottles) are required, but repeat blood cultures should be taken at 12–24-hour intervals if the patient remains septic. There is little convincing evidence to suggest that arterial blood cultures have a higher yield than those taken through a vein[1], unless the infection is caused by an infected arterial line. The source of bacteraemia, if detected, and the causative organisms may vary with the type of ICU, but the respiratory tract and intravascular lines are amongst the commonest sources. However, in a significant proportion of patients, no source is detected.

A local knowledge of causative organisms and recent antimicrobial sensitivity results are helpful in predicting the aetiology, and in guiding empirical therapy[13]. Blood cultures are too often omitted but should be taken and, if necessary, repeated in the acutely ill patient with suspected infection before antibiotics are started or changed. Whilst intravascular lines, including central venous catheters (CVCs), should be strongly suspected as a focus of local or systemic infection, their removal either for diagnostic or therapeutic reasons should be undertaken only after careful consideration. In particular, the policy of routinely replacing CVCs to reduce a perceived high incidence of catheter-related infections should be reviewed[14].

Lower respiratory infections

Ventilator-associated lower respiratory infection remains one of the most important infections acquired in the ICU and together with severe community-acquired pneumonia accounts for considerable mortality. Although there is no single or universally agreed diagnostic approach, there is increasing recognition of the need for BAL, protected brush or protected catheter specimens (i.e. PBS) or non-bronchoscopic lavage to confirm the microbial aetiology and to guide definitive therapy. Pneumonia may be suspected if there have been two or more of the following: two temperature spikes greater than 38.5°C during 24 hours and a raised or depressed white cell count, and three of the following: purulent sputum or tracheal aspirates, new infiltrates on chest X-ray (see Figure 4.5), a rise of 0.15 in FIo_2 to maintain equivalent oxygenation and positive cultures from alveolar secretions, i.e. positive BAL or PBS. Agreed guidelines for the taking and processing of BAL and PBS specimens are now available[15, 16], some of the key aspects of which are:

1. Hypoxia (<70 mmHg on FIo_2 >70%), positive end-expiratory pressure >15 cmH$_2$O, active bronchospasm, recent acute myocardial infarction, unstable arrhythmia, hypotension or thrombocytopenia are relative contra-indications to bronchoscopy.
2. The sampling area for BAL/PBS is based on the location of new or progressive infiltrates on chest X-ray or the presence of purulent secretions seen during bronchoscopy.
3. At least 120 ml are necessary for retrieving secretions from the periphery of the lung and the first aliquot should not be submitted for quantitative bacterial cultures or microscopic evaluation.
4. The Gram stain provides useful information in selecting empirical therapy and the presence of intracellular organisms is a good predictor of ventilator-associated pneumonia.
5. A culture result of >10^4 colony forming units ml^{-1} should be considered significant; a lower level may be significant, however, in the presence of concurrent antibiotics.
6. Additional investigations to exclude less common causes such as *Legionella*, pulmonary aspergillosis and *P. carinii* should be carefully considered in the light of clinical circumstances.

Blood cultures are also indicated to help make a diagnosis and detect bacteraemic pneumonia, which has a poorer prognosis.

CNS infections

It is imperative to diagnose and identify the aetiology of meningitis, encephalitis and brain abscess as soon as possible. Imaging techniques, i.e. CT and

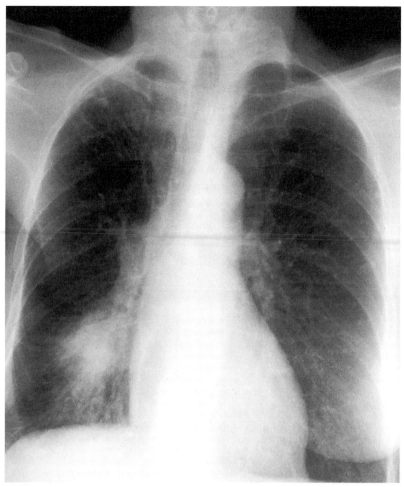

Figure 4.5 Chest X-ray showing segmental consolidation with some atelectasis of the right lateral basal and posterior basal segments.

increasingly MRI, together with the biochemical and microbial analysis of CSF following a lumbar puncture (LP), are the most useful investigations. However, LP is contraindicated if there are localizing signs such as a hemiparesis, or if there is any suggestion of raised intracranial pressure (e.g. papilloedema) on clinical examination, or lateral shift of the midline structures, or obliteration of the fourth ventricle on CT or MRI. Again, blood cultures should usually be performed in any acutely ill patient suspected of having an intracranial infection. The main diagnostic approaches to the three major CNS infections are outlined in Table 4.3.

Table 4.3   Routine laboratory investigations to diagnose CNS infections.

Meningitis	Encephalitis	Brain abscess

CSF
  Biochemistry, microscopy,
  culture and PCR for
  meningococci
	CSF
	  Biochemistry, microscopy,
	  viral culture and PCR for
	  herpes simplex virus
		Pus
		  Microscopy
		  and culture

Other
  Throat swabs for culture,
  petechiae for microscopy
  and blood for serology
  and PCR
	Other
	  Paired blood specimens
	  for viral titres (e.g. Lyme
	  disease and Epstein–Barr
	  virus)
		Other
		  Check ears,
		  sinuses, etc.
		  for primary
		  source

Key points

- Comprehensive clinical assessment is of paramount importance and should guide all laboratory and any other investigations.
- Whilst a raised white cell count may indicate the presence of infection, this test is neither sensitive nor specific enough on its own to suggest infection.
- Plain X-rays and ultrasonography are useful initial imaging investigations.
- Microscopy may provide a rapid presumptive diagnosis but culture of bacteria facilitates antibiotic susceptibility testing, which is important in guiding therapy.
- Antigen detection and molecular methods such as PCR are potentially rapid and useful but to date many of these have either not been clinically validated or are not widely available.
- Blood cultures should be taken in every acutely ill patient in addition to specific investigations such as CSF, BAL, etc.

REFERENCES

1. O'Grady NP, Barie PS, Bartlett J et al. (1998) Practice parameters for evaluating new fever in critically ill adult patients. *Critical Care Medicine* **26**: 392–408.
2. Kirschenbaum LA, Astiz ME, Rackow EC (1998) Interpretation of blood lactate concentrations in patients with sepsis. *Lancet* **352**: 921–922.
3. Byl B, Devière J, Saint-Hubert F et al. (1997) Evaluation of tumour necrosis factor-α, interleukin-6 and C-reactive protein plasma levels as predictors of bacteraemia in patients presenting signs of sepsis without shock. *Clinical Microbiology and Infection* **3**: 306–313.

4. Romano WM, Platt JF (1994) Ultrasound of the abdomen. *Critical Care Clinics* **10**: 297–319.
5. Zingas AP (1994) Computed tomography of the abdomen in the critically ill. *Critical Care Clinics* **10**: 321–339.
6. Davis LP, Fink-Bennett D (1994) Nuclear medicine in the acutely ill patient – II. *Critical Care Clinics* **10**: 383–400.
7. Tompkins LS, Tenover F, Arvin A (1994) New technology in the clinical microbiology laboratory: what you always wanted to know but were afraid to ask. *Journal of Infectious Diseases* **170**: 1068–1074.
8. Gillespie SH (1998) New polymerase chain reaction-based diagnostic techniques for bacterial respiratory infection. *Current Opinion in Infectious Diseases* **11**: 133–138.
9. Klapper PE, Cleator GM (1998) European guidelines for diagnosis and management of patients with suspected herpes simplex encephalitis. *Clinical Microbiology and Infection* **4**: 178–180.
10. Read SJ, Kurtz JB (1999) Laboratory diagnosis of common viral infections in the central nervous system by using a single multiplex PCR screening assay. *Journal of Clinical Microbiology* **37**: 1352–1355.
11. van Burik J-A, Myerson D, Schreckhise RW *et al.* (1998) Panfungal PCR assay for detection of fungal infection in human blood specimens. *Journal of Clinical Microbiology* **36**: 1169–1175.
12. Vannuffel P, Laterre P-F, Bouyer M *et al.* (1998) Rapid and specific molecular identification of methicillin-resistant *Staphylococcus aureus* in endotracheal aspirates from mechanically ventilated patients. *Journal of Clinical Microbiology* **36**: 2366–2368.
13. Crowe M, Ispahani P, Humphreys H *et al.* (1998) Bacteraemia in the adult intensive care unit of a teaching hospital in Nottingham, UK, 1985–1996. *European Journal of Clinical Microbiology and Infectious Diseases* **17**: 377–384.
14. O'Leary M, Bihari D (1998) Central venous catheters – time for change? *British Medical Journal* **316**: 1918–1919.
15. Meduri GU, Chastre J (1992) The standardization of bronchoscopic techniques for ventilator-associated pneumonia. *Chest* **102**: 557S–564S.
16. Baselski VS, El-Torky M, Coalson JJ *et al.* (1992) The standardization of criteria for processing and interpreting laboratory specimens in patients with suspected ventilator-associated pneumonia. *Chest* **102**: 571S–579S.

5 General aspects of management of infection

Management incorporates general and specific aspects of therapy as well as prevention and diagnosis. The prevention of infection is discussed in Chapter 3 but some aspects of this are closely linked with decisions of a therapeutic nature that are discussed below.

The treatment of infection in the acutely ill intensive care unit (ICU) patient involves organ support, removing the focus of infection and appropriate antimicrobial chemotherapy. The risk of death increases by 15–20% with failure of each organ, and this together with delays in the start of antibiotic therapy increases the mortality rate by 10–15%[1], emphasizing the necessity for effective management in acute sepsis.

PREVENTION OF INFECTION

All ICUs should have an infection control policy based on standard principles. Staff should be aware of local patterns of antibiotic resistance as this also helps guide the empirical treatment of suspected infection. The routine culture of the environment and personnel, the use of sticky floor mats and regular decontamination of rooms with disinfectant have no role in routine prevention of infection. The isolation of any new admissions on suspicion of an infectious disease or of any patient suspected of carrying resistant microbes (e.g. methicillin-resistant *Staphylococcus aureus*; MRSA) until microbiological results are available together with the rapid diagnosis and treatment of infection contributes greatly to the control of infection (see Chapter 3).

Antacids and histamine H_2 receptor blockers administered to prevent stress ulceration raise gastric pH, which may facilitate colonization of the airways with potential pathogens. The introduction of sucralfate, a mucosal protective agent with little effect on gastric pH, has reduced the disruption of normal flora and may reduce the consequent risk of nosocomial pneumonia, especially late-onset pneumonia, although this is controversial[2], and more recent evidence suggests that ranitidine may be more effective in reducing significant bleeding[3].

The use of selective decontamination of the digestive tract (SDD) is theoretically attractive as most infections in patients in the ICU are endogenous in origin from the gastrointestinal tract (as discussed in Chapter 3). A combination of non-absorbable antibiotics (polymyxin, tobramycin and amphotericin B) is applied topically to the throat and stomach and thence to the gut to eliminate potential pathogens without affecting the protective anaerobic flora. SDD is usually administered with a systemic antibiotic for a few days until decontamination is effective. This therapy cannot be given concurrently with sucralfate as the latter inactivates the antibiotics. SDD suppresses bacterial overgrowth which is responsible for secondary endogenous infection, translocation and systemic inflammation. Despite reducing secondary infection, SDD is costly, may facilitate the emergence of resistant organisms and, although it has some effect on mortality, its future role remains uncertain[4–7].

EARLY DIAGNOSIS

Diagnosis of infection is often difficult and should be made by reference to strictly applied criteria (see Chapter 4). A multidisciplinary approach, involving intensivists, medical microbiologists/infectious diseases physicians, radiologists, ICU nurses and others, to the diagnosis and management of infection optimizes patient care. Sepsis is especially difficult to diagnose in the postoperative or post-traumatic patient as there may be several other causes for some of the clinical features. Fever occurs in the absence of sepsis with large haematomas or as a complication of blood transfusion, and the white blood cell (WBC) count may be elevated in other inflammatory states. As soon as sepsis is suspected blood, urine, drainage fluid, sputum and any other appropriate specimens should be sent for microscopy, culture and sensitivity and this is an inherent component of the effective management of infection (see Chapter 4). Simple sputum aspiration is often inadequate to provide accurate information on the colonizing/ infecting organism, and quantitative microbiology of bronchoalveolar lavage or a protected catheter specimen is recommended to confirm the diagnosis of pneumonia (see Chapters 4 and 7)[8]. Knowledge of local flora and antibiotic sensitivity patterns are also helpful in guiding initial empirical therapy before laboratory results are available.

REMOVAL OF INFECTED SOURCE

The most important aspect of the management of infection is drainage of pus or necrotic/infected material and delivery of the correct antibiotic(s) at the right dose. Drainage of pus also facilitates obtaining a good-quality specimen to optimize laboratory diagnosis. Wounds may need debriding and abscesses or haematomas require draining. Wounds should be kept dry, well perfused and the patient's nutrition should be maintained to reduce catabolism, which is important for healing. Invasive catheters (e.g. arterial, intra-abdominal) should not be left *in situ* when they are no longer needed and should always be well secured and manipulated only when necessary (see Chapter 9).

Image-guided percutaneous drainage of abscesses is now the procedure of choice (see Chapter 3). The need for drainage rather than antibiotic treatment alone depends upon individual patient circumstances and the ease of aspiration (Figure 5.1).

Percutaneous drainage and operative surgery should be seen as complementary and the decision about which procedure is most appropriate requires

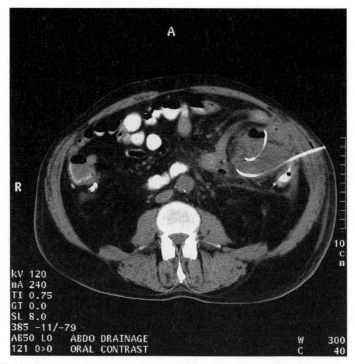

Figure 5.1 Computerized tomography (CT) of an abdominal abscess: the pigtail catheter is shown in the abscess cavity.

collaboration between intensivist, surgeon and radiologist. Percutaneous drainage of an abscess may result in a bacteraemia which may be prevented by antibiotic prophylaxis and by minimizing tissue manipulation. Haemorrhage and perforation of a viscus are, however, possible complications. Most series suggest a 90% success rate for percutaneous drainage – the best results being with unilocular lesions of fluid consistency but viscous fluid and necrotic debris are not easy to drain[9]. Even if an abscess cannot be adequately drained, the condition of the patient may be improved by reducing the 'toxic load' and reducing the need for emergency anaesthesia and surgery[10].

ANTIBIOTICS

Antibiotics kill or inhibit the growth of invading organisms as part of the overall management which includes resuscitation, fluid therapy and the maintenance of oxygen delivery for the prevention of organ failure. There is great anxiety at present about the emergence of resistance organisms, particularly multi-resistant staphylococci and enterococci[11, 12]. Recent reports of the emergence of vancomycin resistance amongst strains of S. aureus, albeit intermediate resistance after prolonged use of vancomycin, are of great concern[13]. The innate capacity of different bacteria to exchange genetic determinants of resistance, especially in the ICU where antibiotic use is high, should encourage greater efforts at infection prevention and more rational antibiotic use. The rapid doubling time of most organisms facilitates the development of several mechanisms of resistance including reduction in cell wall permeability, thus preventing the antibiotic reaching its target, and enzymatic inactivation[14]. It is difficult to differentiate between antibiotic resistance as a marker for patients whose disease puts them at an increased risk of dying from resistance as a *cause* of mortality, as death in the ICU patient is usually due to a variety of factors, only one of which may be an inadequate response to antibiotics[15]. Only a limited number of new classes of antibiotics have been developed and released for clinical use in recent years, hence the anxiety about increasing resistance and the importance of using antibiotics appropriately[16].

As a general rule, patients in the ICU should be given antibiotics only on evidence of a definite infection either to treat an organism of known sensitivity or in a 'best guess' fashion, or in a life-threatening context such as circulatory shock. Otherwise, it is often appropriate to wait and observe if the patient is stable. Among the consequences of inappropriate use in the ICU patient, apart from unnecessary expense, is superinfection, e.g. candidaemia and *Clostridium difficile*-associated diarrhoea.

There are a number of important issues to be considered when prescribing antibiotics (see also Table 5.1). If in doubt, consult a medical microbiologist or infectious diseases physician. Key aspects in the management of infection include:

1. Accurate identification of the organism and its antimicrobial sensitivity is preferable before initiating therapy where possible.
2. The narrowest-spectrum antibiotic to which the organism is sensitive should be used for the shortest period.
3. A bactericidal antibiotic or combination of antibiotics should often be used, particularly in the immunocompromised patients, as bacteriostatic agents depend upon the host defences. Such combinations, e.g. an aminoglycoside with a β-lactam, may also have synergistic effects.
4. The site of infection, route and penetration of the antibiotic should be considered when choosing antibiotics.
5. The likely source of the infection must be assessed.
6. The presence of organ impairment and its effect on metabolism (liver) and excretion (kidney) of the drug must be considered.
7. Drug toxicity and interactions must always be borne in mind.
8. An up-to-date knowledge of locally prevalent organisms and their current sensitivity is of great help in choosing an antibiotic before bacteriological confirmation is available.
9. The dose of an antibiotic will vary according to a number of factors including age, weight, renal function and severity of infection. The prescribing of the so-called 'standard' dose in serious infections may result in failure of treatment but for an antibiotic with a narrow margin between the toxic and therapeutic dose (e.g. an aminoglycoside) it is also important to avoid an excessive dose, and serum concentration monitoring is usually required.

Table 5.1 Key principles of good antimicrobial prescribing in the ICU.

Choice of agents	Antibacterial agents are not indicated for presumed or confirmed viral infections. Consider the likely aetiology and local antimicrobial resistance patterns
Dose	Underdosing rather than overdosing is more common although modifications will be required for renal failure, hepatic failure, dialysis, etc.
Duration	Between 5 and 7 days is adequate for many acute bacterial infections[a] Prolonged therapy (>2 weeks) is costly and leads to resistance and superinfection
Monitoring	Regular serum concentrations are required for aminoglycosides, vancomycin and occasionally for other agents[20–22].

[a] Longer courses are often required for the treatment of *S. aureus* infections.

10. The route of administration of an antibiotic will often depend on the severity of the infection. Life-threatening infections, and therefore most infections in the ICU require intravenous therapy. The duration of the therapy depends on the nature of the infection and the response to treatment.
11. Prescribers should consult the British National Formulary (BNF) or equivalent, or drug data sheets for details of prescribing, including administration regimens; due allowance should be made for individual patient characteristics such as weight, renal or hepatic function. Dose adjustments during haemofiltration are found in recent reviews[17].

In many cases the patient presents initially without an identified pathogen and a choice of antibiotics must be made based on empirical grounds. In these circumstances, a combination of agents that cover a wide range of organisms is preferred. Broad-spectrum coverage should be reviewed as soon as laboratory results become available. The principles of good antimicrobial prescribing in the ICU are similar to those elsewhere in the hospital but the consequences of inappropriate use (e.g. failed therapy and the emergence of resistance) are of greater consequence in seriously ill compromised patients. In the ICU, the commonest reason for prescribing an antibiotic is respiratory infection but many patients receive antibiotics inappropriately, especially cephalosporins, for non-bacterial infection[18].

Classification of antibiotics

Antifungal and antiviral agents are required increasingly in patients in the ICU but antibacterial agents are required most commonly; these generally fall into one of the following categories[19].

Inhibitors of bacterial cell wall synthesis

These include the β-lactams – penicillins, cephalosporins, carbapenems (meropenem) and monobactams such as aztreonam which are bactericidal, and the glycopeptides vancomycin and teicoplanin. β-Lactam agents are relatively non-toxic and allergy to penicillin does not absolutely preclude the use of a cephalosporin or carbapenem, unless there is a history of anaphylaxis or another severe reaction, as the incidence of cross-allergy between penicillins and cephalosporins is only about 10%, and these agents are very effective in the severely ill patient.

Inhibitors of protein synthesis

The majority of these compounds, with the exception of the aminoglycosides, are bacteriostatic at normal doses. This group also includes erythromycin and other macrolides (e.g. clarithromycin), clindamycin, fusidic acid, chloramphenicol and the tetracyclines. The aminoglycosides (i.e. gentamicin, tobramycin, netilmicin, amikacin) are potent anti-Gram-negative antibiotics which are increasingly administered in a single daily dose to achieve rapid killing and to reduce nephrotoxicity and ototoxicity[20, 21]. Drug monitoring is required as the therapeutic index is low with a serious risk of toxicity, and monitoring will help optimize therapy in acutely ill patients[22]. Chloramphenicol, except occasionally for the treatment of meningitis, and the tetracyclines are rarely used in the ICU because less toxic and more effective alternatives are available. Fusidic acid is indicated for the therapy of bone or joint infection but should be combined with another anti-staphylococcal agent; administration by the oral route is less likely to give rise to cholestatic jaundice.

Inhibitors of nucleic acid metabolism

These include the bactericidal quinolones (e.g. ciprofloxacin, ofloxacin, levofloxacin), metronidazole and rifampicin. Quinolones are predominantly active against Gram-negative bacteria and some of these agents have relatively poor activity against Gram-positive pathogens. Rifampicin, an effective anti-mycobacterial agent, is sometimes useful in combination to treat difficult staphylococcal infections such as cerebrospinal fluid (CSF) shunt infections (see Chapter 11). It should, however, never be used alone for this purpose. Further details of these and other antibacterial agents used for both treatment and prophylaxis can be found elsewhere[19, 23–25].

More detailed advice on management of deep *Candida* infection is contained in a number of recently published articles[26, 27] and is discussed further in Chapters 8 and 12.

Empirical antibiotic regimens

What follows are suggested initial antibiotics for the empirical treatment of infection in the ICU (Table 5.2). The information is largely based on what is currently practised in the UK and reflects the antimicrobial susceptibility of the common bacterial pathogens. The choice of one agent over another within a particular drug class (e.g. cefotaxime as an extended-spectrum cephalosporin) is guided by both practice and cost; in other countries an alternative but equivalent agent may be equally efficacious. Gentamicin is included as the amingogylcoside as most bacterial pathogens in the UK remain susceptible, but in other countries amikacin may be preferred due to its susceptibility profile. Listed below are alternative agents within the major drug classes which may be preferred.

Extended-spectrum cephalosporins (instead of cefotaxime):
ceftizoxime, i.v. 1–2 g every 8–12 hours
ceftriaxone, i.v. 2–4 g as a single dose
cefpirome, i.v. 1–2 g every 12 hours

Aminoglycoside (instead of gentamicin):
amikacin, i.v. 15 mg kg^{-1} day^{-1}

Macrolides (instead of erythromycin):
clarithromycin, i.v. 500 mg every 12 hours

Table 5.2 Antibiotic regimens for treatment of infection in the ICU.

Infection	Suggested antibacterial, adult dose	Comment
Respiratory system Community-acquired pneumonia	Cefotaxime, 1–2 g 8-hourly	Twenty per cent of *Streptococcus pneumoniae* and 15% of *Haemophilus influenzae* strains are tetracycline resistant; 15% of *H. influenzae* strains are amoxicillin resistant; pneumococci with decreased penicillin sensitivity are not yet common in the UK
	plus flucloxacillin, 1 g 6-hourly	If *S. aureus* is suspected, e.g. in influenza, measles or aspiration
	plus erythromycin, 0.5–1 g 6-hourly	If *Mycoplasma pneumoniae* or *Legionella pneumophila* infection is suspected
	Consider rifampicin, 0.6 g 12-hourly	If severe *Legionella*

Table 5.2 (Cont'd)

Infection	Suggested antibacterial, adult dose	Comment
ICU-acquired pneumonia	Ceftazidime, 1–2 g 8-hourly *plus* flucloxacillin, 1 g 6-hourly	*S. aureus* and *Pseudomonas aeruginosa* are possible causes
	plus gentamicin, 5 mg kg^{-1} single daily dose	For severe Gram-negative infection; creatinine to be measured within 6 hours of first dose; monitor serum levels
	plus metronidazole, 500 mg 8-hourly	If aspiration is strongly suspected
Pneumocystis carinii pneumonia	(a) Co-trimoxazole, 120 mg kg^{-1} daily in two to four divided doses	Minimum dilution; 1 in 10 in 5% dextrose or 0.9% saline administered over 6 hours Total treatment 3 weeks; can change to oral co-trimoxazole for week 3
	with folinic acid, 15 mg day^{-1} *or*	
	(b) Pentamidine isethionate, 4 mg kg^{-1} over 6 hours	Dilute in 0.9% saline or 5% glucose
	plus prednisolone 40 mg b.i.d. for 7 days, then reduce by 5 mg alternate days	If Pao$_2$ <9.3 kPa
Epiglottitis	Cefotaxime, 1–2 g 8-hourly	*H. influenzae* the most likely bacterial cause but viruses also likely

Table 5.2 (Cont'd)

Infection	Suggested antibacterial, adult dose	Comment
Gastrointestinal system Biliary tract infection	Cefotaxime, 1–2 g 8-hourly *plus* metronidazole, 500 mg 8-hourly *plus* gentamicin 5 mg kg^{-1} single daily dose	For severe Gram-negative infection; measure creatinine within 6 hours of first dose; monitor serum levels
Peritonitis	(a) Cefotaxime, 1–2 g 8-hourly *plus* metronidazole, 500 mg 8-hourly *plus* gentamicin, 5 mg kg^{-1} single dose (b) Piperacillin and tazobactam	*Or* ciprofloxacin, i.v., 400 mg 12-hourly Measure creatinine within 6 hours of first dose; monitor serum levels If recently had cephalosporin antibiotics; gentamicin may be added
Blood Bacteraemia Initial 'blind' therapy	Aminoglycoside *plus* broad-spectrum penicillin *or* a 'third-generation' cephalosporin alone	Choice depends on local resistance patterns and clinical presentation; add metronidazole if anaerobic infection suspected; add flucloxacillin *or* vancomycin if Gram-positive infection is suspected
Community-acquired	(a) Gentamicin, 5 mg kg^{-1} single daily dose *plus* ampicillin, 1 g 4–6-hourly *plus* metronidazole, 500 mg 8-hourly	Measure creatinine within 6 hours of first dose; monitor serum levels *Or* flucloxacillin, 1 g 4–6-hourly

Table 5.2 (Cont'd)

Infection	Suggested antibacterial, adult dose	Comment
Community-acquired (Cont'd)	*or* (b) Cefuroxime, 1.5 g 8-hourly *plus* metronidazole, 500 mg 8-hourly	
Previous antibiotic therapy, severe underlying illness or ICU-acquired	(a) Ceftazidime, 1–2 g 8-hourly *plus* vancomycin, 1 g 12-hourly (*or* teicoplanin, 400 mg 12-hourly × three, reducing to a daily dose of 400 g) *or* (b) Ciprofloxacin, 400 mg 12-hourly *plus* vancomycin, 1 g 12-hourly/ teicoplanin	Monitor vancomycin levels Monitor vancomycin levels
If known to be gastrointestinal associated	Piperacillin/tazobactam, 4.5 g 8-hourly	Monotherapy adequate for gut sepsis
Systemic antiviral agents Herpes encephalitis	Aciclovir, i.v., 10 mg kg^{-1} 8-hourly for 14–21 days	
Chickenpox	As above for 7–10 days	Oral therapy if immunocompetent
Fungal infection Systemic fungal infection	Amphotericin B, up to 1.5 mg kg^{-1} daily or alternative days	Drug of choice; test dose beforehand. Watch for toxicity such as renal impairment, arrhythmias, low potassium or magnesium levels

Table 5.2 (Cont'd)

Infection	Suggested antibacterial, adult dose	Comment
Systemic fungal infection (Cont'd)	*or* AmBisome, 1 mg kg^{-1} day^{-1} increasing to 3 mg kg^{-1} day^{-1} *plus* flucytosine, 200 mg kg^{-1} day^{-1} in four divided doses	Alternative if toxicity arises due to conventional amphotericin B For cryptococcal infection or sensitive isolates of *Candida* spp. Blood levels must be monitored
Proven *Candida albicans* infection	Fluconazole, 400–800 mg daily	2–3 weeks required
Central nervous system Meningitis	Cefotaxime, 2 g 4–6-hourly	Blind therapy
Meningococci	Benzylpenicillin, 2.4 g 4–6-hourly *or* cefotaxime, 2 g 4–6-hourly	Give rifampicin for 2 days (adult 600 mg b.i.d.) before hospital discharge to eradicate carriage
Pneumococci	Cefotaxime, 2 g 4–6-hourly	Requires 10 days treatment; change to benzylpenicillin if susceptibility is confirmed
H. influenzae	Cefotaxime, 2 g 4–6-hourly	Give rifampicin (600 mg once daily) for 4 days before hospital discharge to all close contacts including parents but only if young children in family
Listeria	Ampicillin, 2 g 4-hourly *plus* gentamicin, 5 mg kg^{-1} daily	Measure creatinine within 6 hours of first dose of gentamicin; monitor serum levels

Table 5.2 (Cont'd)

Infection	Suggested antibacterial, adult dose	Comment
Cardiovascular system Native valve endocarditis	Benzylpenicillin, 1–2 g 4-hourly *plus* flucloxacillin, 2 g 4-hourly	Wait for the results of investigations unless life-threatening. Substitute vancomycin, 1 g 12-hourly, or teicoplanin if penicillin allergic
	plus gentamicin, 80–120 mg 8-hourly	Monitor serum levels of gentamicin and vancomycin
Prosthetic valve endocarditis	Vancomycin, 1 g 12-hourly *or* teicoplanin, 400 g 12-hourly × three doses and then 400 mg daily *plus* gentamicin, 80–120 mg 8-hourly	Early consultation with cardiac surgeon essential; monitor serum levels of gentamicin and vancomycin

Antibiotic prophylaxis

Table 5.3. gives a brief overview of antibiotic prophylaxis; more details may be found in local hospital policies or elsewhere[24].

Table 5.3 Antibiotic prophylaxis.

Indication	Antibacterial and dose
Surgical operations on stomach or oesophagus for carcinoma, cholecystectomy in patients with possibly infected bile, and resection of colon and rectum for carcinoma, or in inflammatory bowel disease	Cefuroxime, i.v., 1.5 g plus metronidazole, i.v., 500 mg given 2 hours before operation
Prevention of gas-gangrene in high lower-limb amputations or following major trauma	Benzylpenicillin, i.v., 600 mg every 6 hours for 5 days *or* if penicillin allergic, metronidazole, 500 mg every 8 hours

Table 5.3 (Cont'd)

Indication	Antibacterial and dose
Prevention of meningococcal/ pneumococcal/*Haemophilus* infection following splenectomy or in patients with sickle cell disease	(a) Pneumovax, s.c. or i.m., 0.5 ml, repeat every 5–10 years (b) Hib vaccine: adults require one dose only. The need for reimmunisation is unclear (c) Meningococcal vaccines against group A and C strains, s.c., 0.5 ml. Group A if travelling to endemic areas, group C if recently exposed; this may become routine after its introduction in children (d) Influenza, yearly (e) Permanent antibiotics, especially for the first two years with an oral penicillin (e.g. penicillin V/ 500 mg b.d.) or erythromycin (250 mg b.d.)
Prevention of secondary case of meningococcal meningitis	Rifampicin, 600 mg every 12 hours for 2 days; *for a child*, obtain further advice; ceftriaxone, i.m., 250 mg as a single dose is an alternative in adults or during pregnancy. Contacts of meningitis cases are normally identified to the public or community health authority (e.g. Consultant for Communicable Disease Control in the UK)

Key points

- Within 48 hours of admission to the ICU pathogenic organisms colonize the upper airway and upper gastrointestinal tract.
- All ICUs should have infection control and antibiotic policies.
- The source of infection should be removed wherever possible; this is as important as antibiotic therapy.
- Resistance to antibiotics which may follow inappropriate antibiotic use is more common and of greater consequence in the ICU.
- Antimicrobial treatment must take into account local epidemiology and resistance patterns.

REFERENCES

1. Wheeler AP, Bernard GR (1999) Treating patients with severe sepsis. *New England Journal of Medicine* **340**: 207–214.
2. Prod'hom G, Leuenberger P, Koerfer J et al. (1994) Nosocomial pneumonia in mechanically ventilated patients receiving antacid, ranitidine, or sucralfate as prophylaxis for stress ulcer. *Annals of Internal Medicine* **120**: 653–662.
3. Cook DA, Guyatt G, Marshall J et al. (1998) A comparison of sucralfate and ranitidine for the prevention of upper gastrointestinal bleeding in patients requiring mechanical ventilation. *New England Journal of Medicine* **338**: 791–797.
4. D'Amico R, Pifferi S, Leonetti C et al. (1998) Effectiveness of antibiotic prophylaxis in critically ill adult patients: systematic review of randomised controlled trials. *British Medical Journal* **316**: 1275–1285.
5. Van Saene HKF, Nunn AJ, Petros AJ (1994) Survival benefit by selective decontamination of the digestive tract (SDD). *Infection Control and Hospital Epidemiology* **15**: 443–446.
6. Humphreys H (1994) The future role of selective decontamination of the digestive tract in trauma. *Care of the Critically Ill* **10**: 170–172.
7. Heyland DK (1999) Review of gut-specific strategies to reduce intensive care acquired infections. *Current Opinion in Critical Care* **5**: 132–135.
8. Brun-Buisson C (1993) Microbiological diagnosis of ventilator associated pneumonia: to direct or not to direct sampling. *Intensive Care Medicine* **19**: 367–368.
9. Haaga JR (1990) Imaging, intra-abdominal abscesses and non-operative drainage procedures. *World Journal of Surgery* **14**: 204–209.
10. Schurawitzki H, Karnel F, Stiglbauer R et al. (1992) CT-guided percutaneous drainage and fluid aspiration in intensive care patients. *Acta Radiologica* **33**: 131–136.
11. Michel M, Gutmann L (1997) Methicillin-resistant *Staphylococcus aureus* and vancomycin-resistant enterococci: therapeutic realities and possibilities. *Lancet* **349**: 1901–1906.
12. Schartz MN (1997) Use of antimicrobial agents and drug resistance. *New England Journal of Medicine* **337**: 491–492.
13. Smith TL, Pearson ML, Wilcox KR et al. (1999) Emergence of vancomycin resistance in *Staphylococcus aureus*. *New England Journal of Medicine* **340**: 493–501.
14. Jenkins SG (1990) Mechanisms of bacterial antibiotic resistance. *New Horizons* **4**: 321–332.
15. Solomkin JS (1996) Antimicrobial resistance: an overview. *New Horizons* **4**: 319–320.
16. Standing Medical Advisory Committee Subgroup on Antimicrobial Resistance (1998) *The Path of Least Resistance*. Department of Health, London.
17. Reetze-Bonorden P, Bohler J, Keller E (1993) Drug dosage in patients during continuous renal replacement therapy. *Clinical Pharmacokinetics and Disease Processes* **24**: 362–379.
18. Bergmans DC, Bonten MJ, Gaillard CA et al. (1997) Indications for antibiotic use in ICU patients; a one-year prospective surveillance. *Journal of Antimicrobial Chemotherapy* **39**: 527–535.
19. O'Grady F, Lambert HP, Finch RG et al. (1997) *Antibiotics and Chemotherapy*. Churchill Livingstone, Edinburgh.
20. Cunningham R, Humphreys H (1996) Once-daily gentamicin; translating theory into practice. *European Journal of Clinical Pharmacology* **50**: 151–154.

21. Freeman CD, Nicolau DP, Belliveau PP *et al.* (1997) Once-daily dosing of aminoglycosides; review and recommendations for clinical practice. *Journal of Antimicrobial Chemotherapy* **39**: 677–686.
22. Fraise AP (1998) Monitoring antimicrobials. *Care of the Critically Ill* **14**: 106–108.
23. Simmons NA (1993) Recommendations for endocarditis prophylaxis. *Journal of Antimicrobial Chemotherapy* **31**: 437–438.
24. Timms J, Humphreys H (1997) Antimicrobial prophylaxis in the intensive care unit. *Current Anaesthesia and Critical Care* **8**: 133–138.
25. Working Party of the British Society for Antimicrobial Chemotherapy (1998) Antibiotic treatment of streptococcal, enterococcal and staphylococcal endocarditis. *Heart* **79**: 207–210.
26. Burnie JP (1997) Antibiotic treatment of systemic fungal infections. *Current Anaesthesia and Critical Care* **8**: 180–183.
27. Vincent J-L, Anaissie E, Bruining H *et al.* (1998) Epidemiology, diagnosis and treatment of systemic *Candida* infection in surgical patients under intensive care. *Intensive Care Medicine* **24**: 206–216.

6 Therapeutic interventions in septic shock

INTRODUCTION

The basic treatment of septic shock (Table 6.1) involves administration of oxygen, ventilation and fluid resuscitation, including blood transfusion when required to ensure that blood volume and tissue perfusion are maintained. Vasopressor agents may be required early to restore and maintain tissue oxygenation. Infection must be aggressively sought, treated with the appropriate antibiotics, and any septic source must be surgically drained or removed if possible. Two essential elements should be kept in mind at all times. First, cardiovascular support alone will be ineffective if concurrent treatments to remove the source of sepsis are not employed. Second, clinical assessment and monitoring of the patient's condition at all times are essential to guide therapy. No amount of molecular biology or regionalization of intensive care services will ever replace the need for these fundamental principles of care!

Septic shock is the result of an overwhelming and complex release of inflammatory mediators, causing widespread peripheral vasodilatation and myocardial

Table 6.1 Key points for clinical practice.

Control of infection	Antibiotic therapy Removal of the source if possible – surgical drainage, percutaneous drainage, etc.
Oxygenation	Oxygen administration Mechanical ventilation if required
Haemodynamic resuscitation	Fluid therapy (including blood) – under control of cardiac filling pressures Vasopressor therapy – initial drug is dopamine, but noradrenaline may be also required Inotropic therapy to increase oxygen delivery to the tissues – dobutamine is the preferred agent
Immunotherapy	Only experimental (nothing currently clinically available)

depression (see Chapter 1). The resultant haemodynamic alterations typically include a fall in blood pressure, an increase in cardiac output, and a fall in systemic vascular resistance. Oxygen needs are increased by the inflammatory response, and oxygen extraction capabilities altered by peripheral abnormalities associated with maldistribution of blood flow. Sepsis also induces myocardial depression, through the release of myocardial depressants, the development of myocardial oedema, and alterations in myocardial cell function. Myocardial contractility may be reduced even in the presence of normal or high cardiac output. Thus, despite an increase in cardiac output, oxygen availability to the cell may still be insufficient to meet tissue needs, leading to tissue hypoxia and multiple organ failure. Effective cardiovascular support therefore plays an essential role in the management of the patient with septic shock. The primary aims must be, first, to control the vasodilatation and restore a minimal tissue perfusion pressure and, second, to maintain cardiac function to provide sufficient oxygen transport to the cells (see Figure 6.1).

Although most therapeutic interventions usually lead to an increase in oxygen consumption, reducing oxygen demand may also contribute to a restoration of the equilibrium between oxygen requirement and supply. Thus the early use of mechanical ventilation should be considered, not only to improve gas exchange but also to reduce the oxygen demand of the respiratory muscles. Hyperventilation is common in severe sepsis and can be exacerbated by the need for compensation of the metabolic acidosis or the development of respiratory failure. The resulting increase in the work of breathing can contribute significantly to the increase in the oxygen demand of the body. Finally, current understanding of the pathophysiology of this devastating disease process, and its frequent sequel multi-organ failure (MOF), has also highlighted the need to maintain adequate regional perfusion and oxygenation in these patients.

HAEMODYNAMIC ASSESSMENT

In view of the importance of adequate oxygen balance in ongoing disease, and the need to avoid harmful excessive vasoconstriction, assessment of the haemodynamic status of a septic patient must combine standard haemodynamic parameters, including blood pressure and cardiac output, with measures of tissue oxygenation, including mixed venous oxygen saturation (Sv_{O_2}) and blood lactate concentrations. Cardiac output alone is an inadequate measure of haemodynamic status as it may be normal or even high in septic patients. In the absence of anaemia and hypoxaemia, Sv_{O_2} reflects the relationship between oxygen uptake and cardiac output. Although a normal Sv_{O_2} does not guarantee adequate tissue perfusion, a low Sv_{O_2} is an alarm signal regarding poor tissue oxygenation. Blood lactate levels have been shown to correlate with outcome from septic shock particularly when measured repeatedly[1]. Other possible causes of hyperlactataemia must be excluded; actual levels reflect a balance between production and elimination. Sv_{O_2} and blood lactate levels can only yield information on global oxygenation and yet a patient who appears

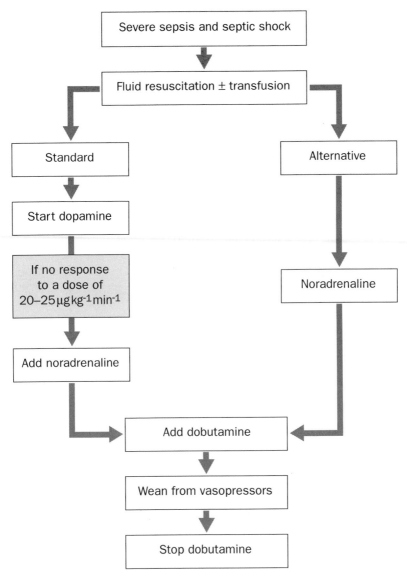

Figure 6.1 Stepwise cardiovascular support in septic shock.

fully resuscitated may have areas of residual regional ischaemia[2]. The use of gastric tonometry to measure gastric intramucosal pH (pHi) or simply the intramucosal carbon dioxide pressure ($Pgco_2$) enables a more regional measure of organ blood flow. A low pHi in patients with septic shock has been associated with a poor outcome and the combination of blood lactate levels with pHi may provide even more valuable information[3]. Importantly, none of these parameters should be considered in isolation but evaluated together in combination with a full clinical assessment.

RESTORING TISSUE PERFUSION PRESSURE

Fluid resuscitation

Uncorrected and persistent hypovolaemia is likely to result in organ failure and death. Increasing cardiac filling pressures excessively may result in worsening pulmonary oedema, but this is better than allowing hypovolaemia and compromising tissue oxygenation. It is difficult to define an optimal level for cardiac filling pressures in the septic patient. Accordingly, a fluid challenge technique, studying the haemodynamic changes induced by a rapid infusion at a rate of 500–1000 ml hour^{-1}, is recommended.

The choice of fluid is still controversial. Many prefer the use of colloids over crystalloids in septic shock, despite their higher price. They have the advantage of remaining in the intravascular space for longer than the equivalent volume of crystalloid. This has two potential effects. Firstly, smaller volumes have to be administered to achieve a given effect, thereby restoring oxygen transport to the cells more rapidly. Secondly, colloid fluids are less likely to promote the development of oedema. Clinical trials have, however, failed to show any superiority of one type of fluid over another, probably because the amount of fluid matters much more than the type.

Red cells must be transfused as required. Some reduction in haematocrit may occur in the absence of bleeding, reflecting the vasodilatation occurring with expansion of the plasma volume. Although the optimal haematocrit in sepsis has not been well defined, maintenance of the haematocrit between 30 and 35%, or the haemoglobin level between 10 and 11 g dl^{-1} is generally agreed. Fluid administration alone restores haemodynamic stability in 30–40% of septic patients who develop arterial hypotension. As may be expected, the prognosis is better in these patients than in those requiring inotropic support.

Vasoactive agents

The effects of the commonly used adrenergic agents are summarized in Table 6.2. Patients who do not respond sufficiently to fluid resuscitation will require vasoactive agents to restore a minimal perfusion pressure. The required pressure is generally considered to be a systolic pressure of 90–100 mmHg, or a mean arterial pressure of 70–75 mmHg.

Dopamine is a naturally occurring amine, the natural precursor of noradrenaline. Its effects are very dose dependent. At low to moderate doses (up to around 10 μg kg^{-1} min^{-1}), β-adrenergic effects predominate, so that the increase in myocardial contractility and the lack of significant vasoconstriction maintain cardiac output. At higher doses (>10 μg kg^{-1} min^{-1}), α-adrenergic effects predominate, resulting in marked vasoconstriction with a greater rise in blood pressure. At very low doses (<2 μg kg^{-1} min^{-1}), dopamine also activates dopaminergic receptors, and this effect may be expected to increase blood flow to the renal parenchyma and splanchnic regions more than to other regions. This pharmacological action has, however, not been demonstrated to be beneficial in critically ill patients.

Table 6.2 Effects of the principal adrenergic agents on the adrenergic receptors.

Agent	Receptor				
	β-Adrenergic		α-Adrenergic	Dopaminergic	
	1	2	1	1	2
Isoprenaline	+++	+++	0	0	0
Dopexamine	+	+++	0	++	+
Dobutamine	+++	+	+	0	0
Dopamine	++	+	++	+++	++
Adrenaline	+++	+++	+++	0	0
Noradrenaline	+++	0	+++	0	0
Phenylephrine	0	0	+++	0	0

+++, major activity; ++, significant activity; +, some activity, 0, no activity.

If hypotension is very severe, another agent with stronger vasopressor properties should be used (or added), and noradrenaline is usually preferred for this purpose. Noradrenaline is an endogenous catecholamine released by terminal nerve endings and secreted by the adrenal medulla. It is a potent α-agonist with moderate β_1 and minimal β_2 activity. It therefore induces peripheral vasoconstriction with a resultant rise in blood pressure, although cardiac output may still be maintained, especially with lower doses.

Several studies have argued the beneficial effects of noradrenaline over dopamine in the septic patient, based on the reasoning that systemic vascular resistance is typically reduced so that the restoration of vascular tone may be beneficial to the organs. Noradrenaline may increase systemic vascular resistance while maintaining cardiac and urine output[4]. Marik and Mohedin found that in 20 septic patients dopamine caused a fall in gastric pHi levels suggesting a decrease in mucosal oxygen availability, whilst noradrenaline caused a rise in gastric pHi, indicating improved gastric tissue oxygenation[5]. Noradrenaline may be most beneficial in conditions of cardiovascular collapse, but once minimal tissue perfusion is restored there is no good evidence that increasing systemic vascular resistance further can result in any clinical improvement. The major risk is to reduce blood flow by excessive vasoconstriction and many therefore administer dobutamine simultaneously to maintain blood flow, and a currently recommended stepwise protocol is shown in Figure 6.1[6].

Adrenaline may also be used in septic shock in those patients who fail to respond to dopamine, and in some centres is used as a substitute for dopamine because it is cheaper. It may, however, induce more tachyarrhythmias and decrease splanchnic perfusion[7]. Hence, the authors do not believe adrenaline is the drug of choice, and its use should be reserved for extreme cases close to cardiopulmonary resuscitation.

As well as acting to restore a minimal tissue perfusion pressure, there is evidence that adrenergic agents may have an anti-inflammatory role to play in septic patients. Van der Poll et al. observed that β-adrenergic stimulation with noradrenaline, adrenaline or isoprenaline inhibited the endotoxin-induced release of tumour necrosis factor (TNF) and interleukin 6 (IL-6) in whole blood ex vivo, while α-adrenergic stimulation had no effect on endotoxin-induced cytokine release[8]. These effects appear to be at least in part due to augmented IL-10 release[9].

IMPROVING REGIONAL BLOOD FLOW

The effects of inotropes on regional blood flow, particularly renal and splanchnic flow, have stimulated particular interest as the importance of local tissue hypoxia in the pathophysiology of multi-organ failure (MOF) has become apparent.

Renal flow
Low-dose dopamine has been widely used in critically ill patients, for its renal-sparing effects but there is in fact little evidence that it has any specific beneficial effect on renal blood flow[10].

Splanchnic flow
The gut is particularly sensitive to alterations in regional blood flow because of the countercurrent mechanism delivering oxygen to the tip of the villi. Gut ischaemia has been associated with the perpetuation of the systemic inflammatory response and hence MOF[11]. The use of gastric tonometry may enable more effective assessment of the effects of various catecholamines on gastric blood flow but the data available are often conflicting, confusing and difficult to interpret. Several studies in septic patients have shown improved hepatosplanchnic blood flow with dopamine but none has consistently shown an improvement in pHi, suggesting that dopamine may redistribute flow away from the gastric mucosa[7, 12, 13]. There is some evidence to suggest dopamine may hasten the development of gut ischaemia[14]. Dopexamine may have beneficial effects on hepatosplanchnic blood flow in septic patients but its effects on pHi have not been consistent[15]. Noradrenaline has variable effects on pHi and hepatosplanchnic blood flow[5, 7, 16], and adrenaline may be deleterious[17]. Overall, dobutamine is the inotrope that seems most consistently to improve hepatosplanchnic blood flow and pHi[12, 18].

It may be preferable to tailor therapy according to a number of criteria presented in Table 6.3. Obviously clinical evaluation remains very important, but

Table 6.3   Assessment of oxygen availability.

Assessment	Criteria

Clinical	Arterial hypotension
	Signs of hypoperfusion
	   Altered mental status
	   Oliguria
	   Altered skin perfusion

Derived	Low mixed venous oxygen saturation (Svo_2 <65%) Hyperlactataemia (blood lactate >2 mmol l^{-1})

Under investigation	Tonometry – decreased gastric intramucosal pH
	   (<7.32), raised intramucosal Pco_2
	   (>6 mmHg above $Paco_2$)
	Tissue Po_2 electrodes
	Near infrared spectroscopy

this alone may not be sufficient. In complex cases, the demonstration of oxygen consumption rate versus delivery (Vo_2/Do_2) interdependency may be informative. The use of a cardiac index/oxygen extraction diagram may be useful for this purpose[19].

IMPROVING TISSUE OXYGEN EXTRACTION

Whilst restoring an adequate oxygen supply to the tissues is essential, the ability to improve oxygen extraction would also be beneficial. The role of nitric oxide (NO) in septic shock is well documented but it does not appear to contribute to altered oxygen extraction. N-acetyl-L-cysteine (NAC), an oxygen free radical scavenger, was shown to improve oxygen extraction capabilities in a study of patients with septic shock[20]. The lazaroid tirilizad mesylate has also been shown to improve oxygen extraction capabilities in a dog model[21]. Both these agents were shown to have beneficial effects on myocardial function. However, the use of such agents remains experimental at present.

INCREASING MYOCARDIAL CONTRACTILITY

Adrenergic agents

Myocardial depression can limit the oxygen supply to the tissues even when cardiac output is normal or high. An inotropic agent without vasoconstrictive properties is necessary to improve contractility. Dobutamine has become the agent of choice. It is a synthetic catecholamine with selective β_1-adrenergic effects. It mediates an increase in myocardial contractility with no increase in mean arterial pressure or heart rate. The effect of adding dobutamine at doses of $5\,\mu g\,kg^{-1}\,min^{-1}$ to a standard resuscitation regimen in patients with septic shock caused a marked increase in cardiac index and increased oxygen uptake (Vo_2) and oxygen delivery (Do_2)[6]. Other studies support an improvement in gastric blood flow with dubutamine infusion[22]. Dobutamine can also enable the administration of larger amounts of intravenous fluids than dopamine by a reduced effect on cardiac filling pressures[23]. The dose of dobutamine is hard to quantify as it is difficult to define optimal levels of cardiac output and Do_2. Sequential blood lactate levels are of use, as a fall in blood lactate concentration can reflect an improvement in tissue perfusion[1], but they are too imprecise to guide therapy directly.

Dopexamine is a newer synthetic agent combining strong β-adrenergic and dopaminergic effects with no α effects. Comparing dobutamine and dopexamine infusion in endotoxin-treated dogs, the systemic vascular resistance decreased more with dopexamine, but cardiac output and Do_2 increased with both substances with no effect on mean arterial pressure[24]. Dopexamine use is limited by significant tachycardia which can occur at a higher infusion rate. The dopaminergic effects of dopexamine are weaker than those of dopamine, but overall the effect is to increase splanchnic blood flow. Low doses of dopexamine may therefore be a useful alternative to low-dose dopamine for increasing hepatosplanchnic blood flow.

Phosphodiesterase inhibitors

Phosphodiesterase inhibitors have positive inotropic and vasodilating effects. The combination of a phosphodiesterase inhibitor with adrenergic agents should obtain additive inotropic effects on the myocardium whilst cancelling out peripheral effects. Their use has not been widely studied in septic shock but they have been found to increase cardiac output in cardiogenic shock. Amrinone infusion in endotoxin-treated dogs was found to increase cardiac output, oxygen transport and oxygen consumption whilst having no effect on systemic hypotension, although lowering systemic vascular resistance[25].

IMMUNOTHERAPEUTIC AGENTS

Advances in immunology and molecular biology during the 1990s revealed that the host's inflammatory response to infection contributes substantially to the development of septic shock[26, 27]. Attempts to identify a single central mediator of the disease have been unconvincing to date. It seems more likely that the development of sepsis is related to a complex interplay between pro- and anti-inflammatory mediators, many of which have now been identified, thus facilitating experimentation with a whole new range of therapies (Table 6.4). The sepsis cascade is often initiated by the release of endotoxin and/or other microbiological metabolites into the circulation (see Chapter 1). This prompts the release of TNFα, IL-1, IL-6, IL-8 and platelet-activating factor (PAF) by mononuclear phagocytes and endothelial cells. After these initial releases, arachidonic acid is metabolized to form leukotrienes, thromboxane A_2 and prostaglandins. IL-1 and IL-6 activate the T cells to produce further cytokines, including granulocyte colony-stimulating factor (G-CSF)[28].

Table 6.4 Potential immunomodulatory interventions in sepsis.

Target	Intervention
Endotoxin	Polyclonal immunoglobulins J5 antiserum Monoclonal antibodies to lipid A: H1A1, E5 Soluble CD14 High-density lipoproteins, chylomicrons Bactericidal permeability-increasing protein Cationic antimicrobial protein (CAP18) Antibodies to CD14 Taurolidine Endotoxin-neutralizing protein Polymyxin conjugates (haemoperfusion, dextran) Lipopolysaccharide antagonists (ENP, E5531, B464) Tyrosine kinase inhibitors Lipid A analogues: lipid X, B464, mono- and diphosphoryl lipid A
TNF	Anti-TNF antibodies: murine, FAB2 fragments, humanized Soluble TNF receptors P55 and P75 Thalidomide
Interferon γ	Interferon γ Antibodies to interferon γ
IL-1	IL-1 receptor antagonist (IL-Ira) Anti-IL-1 antibodies Soluble IL-1 receptors
cAMP	Prostaglandin E1 Pentoxifylline Adrenergic agents Amrinone
Complement	C1 esterase inhibitor Antibodies to C5a

Table 6.4 (Cont'd)

Target	Intervention
Bradykinin	Bradykinin receptor antagonists
Adhesion molecules	Antibodies to CD11/CD18 and E-selectins
Proteases	Antiprotease
PLA_2	PLA_2 antagonists
PAF	PAF antagonists
Arachidonic acid metabolites	Ibuprofen, indomethacin Lipoxygenase inhibitor Leukotriene receptor antagonists Chloroquine
Nitric oxide	Nitric oxide synthase antagonists (L-NMMA, L-NAME) Methylene blue
Oxygen free radicals	N-acetylcysteine, procysteine Superoxide dismutase catalase Dapsone, desferrioxamine Vitamins E and C, selenium
Coagulation factors	Antithrombin, protein C
Cytokine removal	Haemofiltration techniques
Immunostimulation	G-CSF
Various	Melanotonin PGG-glucan Immunonutrition, glutamine, α-ketoglutamate Corticosteroids, 21 aminosteroids IL-10 Calcium entry blockers

cAMP, cyclic adenosine monophosphate; L-NMMA, L-N-monomethyl-arginine; L-NAME, L-N-arginine methyl ester; G-CSF, granulocyte colony-stimulating factor; PLA_2, phospholipase A_2; PAF, platelet-activating factor; TNF, tumour necrosis factor; PGG, poly([1–6]β-D-glucopyranosyl-[1–3]β-D-glucopyranose).

Whilst it has been possible to identify a network of mediator release, identifying the exact role of each of them is difficult. One problem is that these mediators may have beneficial, as well as deleterious, effects; in particular, an immunological response is very desirable in response to moderate infection. Another complication is that of varying cellular receptivity to stimuli. Finally, it seems that the mediators of septic shock interact with one another in very complex ways so that even if one pathway of the network is denied, mediator release may be facilitated via another. Indeed, it has been suggested that the number of interactions between mediators may approximate the number of mediators squared[29]. This indicates that a combination therapy, rather than blocking a single mediator, is most likely to offer an effective defence against septic shock. A few of the 'key players' in septic shock are presented here with the hope of elucidating as best as is possible the various therapeutic options available for the future.

Endotoxins

It is very likely that the endotoxin-evoked inflammatory response is an important weapon in the host's initial defence against infection. However, persistent or repetitive inflammatory provocation may lead to an 'anarchic' situation, in which the body can no longer control its own inflammatory response, resulting in endothelial damage, interstitial oedema and altered organ function[29]; the risk of MOF is high.

Endotoxins occur primarily as lipopolysaccharide (LPS) components of the outer membrane of Gram-negative bacteria and are an extremely potent trigger of the network of mediators and the complement cascade. The endotoxin molecule consists of an outer layer of structurally and antigenically diverse oligosaccharides and a core of similarly structured oligosaccharides. Bound to this core is lipid A which has a highly conserved structure and is responsible for most of the toxicity of endotoxin. Two monoclonal antibodies directed at core LPS and lipid A have been developed: E5, a murine monoclonal IgM antibody, and HA-1A, a human monoclonal antibody, but initially promising results could not be confirmed[30, 31].

Another anti-endotoxin approach is the possibility of using the naturally occurring molecule known as bactericidal permeability-increasing protein (BPI). This occurs in the polymorphonuclear leukocytes and, although not an antibody, binds very strongly with lipid A to inhibit the toxicity of endotoxin. Recombinant BPI has been shown to protect against fatal doses of endotoxin in animals; studies in human severe meningococcal sepsis showed an improvement in outcome and a phase III trial is currently underway[32].

Tumour necrosis factor

Much attention has been focused on TNFα, since it has several characteristics consistent with being a central mediator of septic shock:

1. High blood levels of TNFα are found in patients with a high probability of death or organ failure[33].

2. Administration of TNF in animals leads to septic shock and organ failure[34]. Administration of TNF in volunteers leads to similar effects as those associated with endotoxin infection[35].
3. Administration of TNF antibodies in animals can protect against the administration of endotoxin and live bacteria[36].

TNF is also incriminated in myocardial depression via several mechanisms, including the development of myocardial oedema, alterations in the myocardial cell membrane or in the contractile apparatus. Clinical studies have concentrated on the effect of blocking TNFα with antibodies in septic shock patients. A recently conducted international multicentre placebo-controlled trial of a murine anti-TNF antibody failed, however, to show an improvement in outcome[37].

Research is also being undertaken in the field of naturally occurring soluble receptors to TNF. A recent study presented worrying results, however. A phase II, blinded, randomized trial, of either a placebo or recombinant human dimeric TNF receptor p75, suggested a worse outcome in the treated group. These results raise serious concerns about the potential harmful consequences of anticytokine therapies in sepsis and septic shock.

Interleukin 1

IL-1 is a pro-inflammatory mediator produced by various cell types in response to endotoxin and other stimuli. IL-1 binds to two tissue receptors, type I found primarily on T cells and hepatocytes, and type II found predominantly on B cells, neutrophils and bone marrow precursor cells. Injection of IL-1 into animals results in fever, neutrophilia, hypotension and the features of septic shock. IL-1 does not appear to be as potent as TNF, but an important synergism exists between the two mediators, with IL-1 potentiating the effects of TNFα[38]. Experimentally IL-1, like TNF, has been implicated in the pathogenesis of sepsis-induced myocardial depression[39].

IL-1 receptor antagonist (IL-1ra) is a naturally occurring substance produced at the same time and by the same stimuli as IL-1, but in larger amounts. It recognizes and binds to both types of IL-1 receptor but has no IL-1 agonist activity. Once bound, it inhibits IL-1 binding thus providing the body with a protective mechanism against the harmful effects of IL-1. In animal models of septic shock, recombinant IL-1ra has been shown to reduce mortality and to improve cardiovascular performance[40]. An initial trial in patients with septic shock showed an apparent dose-related reduction in mortality[41], but this has not been confirmed[42].

Platelet-activating factor

The phospholipid mediator PAF can be produced by cytokines as well as macrophages, neutrophils, eosinophils, endothelial cells and platelets. Raised levels of PAF have been detected in endotoxin-induced hypotension and endotoxin-induced lung injury in rats[43]. The effects of TNF have been shown to be markedly reduced in the absence of PAF[44]. PAF can alter the vascular tone and permeability as well as exerting a negative inotropic effect on the heart which may contribute to a decrease in arterial blood pressure. Recent randomized clinical trials of PAF antagonists in severe sepsis failed, however, to show an improvement in outcome[45].

Oxygen free radicals

Oxygen free radicals are highly reactive agents which may be produced by the enzymes of activated granulocytes and macrophages. In particular peroxide and hydroxyl radicals are responsible for endothelial damage and oedema. Oxygen free radicals have also been implicated in myocardial depression of sepsis, and inactivation of the α_1-proteinase inhibitor, thus promoting the destructive action of liberated proteinases. The augmentation of vascular permeability by oxygen free radicals implicates them in the mediation of acute respiratory distress syndrome (ARDS)[46].

Of a number of therapeutic options, N-acetylcysteine and procysteine are the most promising. Such agents are particularly attractive because they can augment the oxygen extraction capabilities in septic shock and improve haemodynamic performance[47].

Nitric oxide

The constitutional synthesis of nitric oxide via the endothelial cells is calcium dependent and has an important role in physiological vasodilatation and neurotransmission. Mediators of septic shock such as TNF and endotoxin can, however, induce the calcium-independent synthase enzyme which is thought to be responsible for the decrease in arterial pressure associated with septic shock. Nitric oxide has also been implicated in sepsis-induced myocardial depression and is thought to have direct cytotoxic effects leading to tissue injury and organ failure[48, 49]. There is a possibility that nitric oxide synthesis inhibitors may increase survival rates in septic shock by increasing mean arterial pressure and reducing cytotoxic damage. The use in humans of nitric oxide synthase (NOS) inhibitors, e.g. L-N-monomethyl-arginine (L-NMMA), has been shown transiently to increase arterial pressure, allowing a reduction in the dose of vasopressor agents. This increase has been at the expense of a drop in cardiac output and tissue perfusion[50]. It may also selectively reduce hepatosplanchnic blood flow and its use remains experimental. More selective NOS blockade may provide a more promising treatment but no agent has yet been shown to be beneficial.

An alternative method of blocking nitric oxide production is to inhibit guanylate cyclase by the use of methylene blue. In experimental studies in a model of endotoxic sepsis, methylene blue produced an increase in splanchnic blood flow[51]. Clinical studies in patients with septic shock demonstrated an increase in mean arterial pressure[52]. However, no overall benefit in patient outcome or oxygen transport was demonstrated.

Corticosteroids

Corticosteroids are potent anti-inflammatory agents acting chiefly through the inhibition of phospholipase A_2, the enzyme responsible for the generation of arachidonic acid metabolites and PAF. Corticosteroids also inhibit the activation of the complement cascade and the synthesis of $TNF\alpha$ and IL-1, and have been shown to inhibit the induction of NOS by endotoxin[53]. The latter mechanism may explain why corticosteroids have been found to be effective when administered before or very early during the septic challenge and why this efficiency is lost when the administration takes place later as a therapeutic intervention.

Previously, large, double-blinded, randomized, multicentre studies have failed to demonstrate any beneficial effect of corticosteroid administration in either septic patients or those with ARDS[54, 55]. A recent study of 41 patients with septic shock requiring catecholamines, however, demonstrated that modest doses of hydrocortisone in patients with shock for more than 96 hours resulted in a significant improvement in haemodynamics and survival[56]. This study, which needs to be repeated in larger numbers of patients, may be indicating that there is a narrow dose range in which corticosteroids have a beneficial effect.

Granulocyte colony-stimulating factor

G-CSF is a potent stimulator of the neutrophilic immunological response. Whereas many of the treatments so far discussed have looked at ways of blocking this response, G-CSF treatment aims to increase it. In an animal model of sepsis, administration of G-CSF was associated with prolonged survival times, improved arterial blood pressure and improved cardiac function[57]. Clearance of endotoxin was also noted. In patients with septic shock, stimulating an already anarchic immune response is possibly unwise; however, this treatment may prove successful either in fortifying a patient once a stable condition has been restored and/or as a prophylactic measure in high-risk surgical patients[58]. Studies in septic shock are awaited.

Key points

- The inflammatory response results in profound vasodilatation and myocardial depression.
- Blood pressure falls, cardiac output increases and systemic vascular resistance is reduced.
- Maintenance of tissue oxygenation is a fundamental goal of treatment.
- Diagnosis and eradication of the source of sepsis must accompany antibiotic therapy.
- Cardiovascular support starts with fluid resuscitation before administration of inotropes under haemodynamic monitoring.
- Immunomodulation, although theoretically attractive, has yet to show therapeutic advantages.

REFERENCES

1. Bakker J, Gris P, Coffernils M *et al.* (1996) Serial blood lactate levels can predict the development of multiple organ failure following septic shock. *American Journal of Surgery* **171**: 221–226.
2. Fiddian-Green RG, Haglund U, Gutierrez G *et al.* (1993) Goals for the resuscitation of shock. *Critical Care Medicine* **21**: S25–S31.
3. Friedman G, Berlot G, Kahn RJ *et al.* (1995) Combined measurements of blood lactate concentrations and gastric intramucosal pH in patients with severe sepsis. *Critical Care Medicine* **23**: 1184–1193.
4. Martin C, Papazian L, Perrin G *et al.* (1993) Norepinephrine or dopamine for the treatment of hyperdynamic septic shock? *Chest* **103**: 1826–1831.
5. Marik PE, Mohedin J (1994) The contrasting effects of dopamine and norepinephrine on systemic and splanchnic oxygen utilization in hyperdynamic sepsis. *Journal of the American Medical Association* **272**: 1354–1357.
6. Vincent JL, Roman A, Kahn RJ (1990) Dobutamine administration in septic shock: addition to a standard protocol. *Critical Care Medicine* **18**: 689–693.
7. Meier-Hellmann A, Reinhart K (1994) Influence of catecholamines on regional perfusion and tissue oxygenation in septic shock patients. In: *Sepsis. Current Perspectives in Pathophysiology and Therapy* (eds Reinhart K, Eyrick K, Sprung C), pp 274–291. Springer, Berlin.
8. Van der Poll T, Jansen J, Endert E *et al.* (1994) Noradrenaline inhibits lipopolysaccharide-induced tumor necrosis factor and interleukin 6 production in human whole blood. *Infection and Immunology* **62**: 2046–2050.
9. Van der Poll T, Coyle SM, Barbosa K *et al.* (1996) Epinephrine inhibits tumor necrosis factor-α and potentiates interleukin 10 production during human endotoxemia. *Journal of Clinical Investigation* **97**: 713–719.
10. Vincent JL (1994) Renal effects of dopamine: may our dream ever come true? *Critical Care Medicine* **22**: 5–6.
11. Meakins JL, Marshall JC (1989) The gut as the motor of multiple system organ failure. In: *Splanchnic Ischemia and Multiple Organ Failure* (eds Marston A, Buckley GB, Fiddian-Green R), pp 339–348. Edward Arnold, London.
12. Neviere R, Mathieu D, Chagnon JL *et al.* (1996) The contrasting effects of dobutamine and dopamine on gastric mucosal perfusion in septic patients. *American Journal of Respiratory and Critical Care Medicine* **154**: 1684–1688.
13. Meier-Hellmann A, Bredle DL, Specht M *et al.* (1997) The effects of low-dose dopamine on splanchnic blood flow and oxygen uptake in patients with septic shock. *Intensive Care Medicine* **23**: 31–37.
14. Segal JM, Phang T, Walley KR (1992) Low-dose dopamine hastens onset of gut ischemia in a porcine model of hemorrhagic shock. *Journal of Applied Physiology* **73**: 1159–1164.
15. Smithies M, Yee TH, Jackson L *et al.* (1994) Protecting the gut and the liver in the critically ill: effects of dopexamine. *Critical Care Medicine* **22**: 789–795.
16. Zhang H, Smail N, Cavral A *et al.* (1997) Effects of norepinephrine on regional blood flow and oxygen extraction capabilities during endotoxic shock. *American Journal of Respiratory and Critical Care Medicine* **155**: 1965–1971.
17. Levy B, Bollaert PE, Charpentier C *et al.* (1997) Comparison of norepinephrine and dobutamine to epinephrine for hemodynamics, lactate metabolism, and gastric tonometric variables in septic shock. *Intensive Care Medicine* **23**: 282–287.

18. Gutierrez G, Clark C, Brown SD *et al.* (1994) Effect of dobutamine on oxygen consumption and gastric mucosal pH in septic patients. *American Journal of Respiratory and Critical Care Medicine* **150**: 324–329.

19. Vincent JL, Silance PG, De Backer D (1994) The cardiac index/oxygen extraction diagram to assess hemodynamic status. In: *Yearbook in Intensive Care and Emergency Medicine* – 1994 (ed. Vincent JL), pp 144–151. Springer, Berlin.

20. Spies CD, Reinhart K, Witt I *et al.* (1994) Influence of *N*-acetylcysteine on indirect indicators of tissue oxygenation in septic shock patients: results from a prospective, randomised, double-blind study. *Critical Care Medicine* **22**: 1738–1746.

21. Zhang H, Spapen H, Manikis P *et al.* (1995) Tirilazad mesylate (U74006F) inhibits effects of endotoxin in dogs. *American Journal of Physiology* **268**: H1847–H1855.

22. Silverman HJ, Tuma P (1992) Gastric tonometry in patients with sepsis. Effects of dobutamine infusions and packed red blood cell transfusions. *Chest* **102**: 184–188.

23. Vincent JL, Van der Linden P, Domb M *et al.* (1987) Dopamine compared with dobutamine in experimental septic shock: relevance to fluid administration. *Anesthesia and Analgesia* **66**: 565–571.

24. Preiser JC, Armistead CW, Le Minh T *et al.* (1989) Increase in oxygen supply during experimental septic shock: the effects of dobutamine versus dopexamine. *Journal of Critical Care* **4**: 40–44.

25. De Boelpaepe C, Vincent JL, Contempre B *et al.* (1989) Combination of norepinephrine and amrinone in the treatment of endotoxin shock. *Journal of Critical Care* **4**: 202–207.

26. Dinarello CA, Wolff SM (1993) The role of interleukin 1 in disease [published erratum appears in *New England Journal of Medicine* **328**: 744]. *New England Journal of Medicine* **328**: 106–113.

27. Nathan C, Sporn M (1991) Cytokines in context. *Journal of Cell Biology* **113**: 981–986.

28. Jacobs RF, Tabor DR (1989) Immune cellular interactions during sepsis and septic injury. *Critical Care Clinics* **5**: 9–26.

29. Bone RC (1991) The pathogenesis of sepsis. *Annals of Internal Medicine* **115**: 457–469.

30. McCloskey RV, Straube RC, Sanders C *et al.* (1994) Treatment of septic shock with human monoclonal antibody HA-1A. A randomized, double-blind, placebo-controlled trial. *Annals of Internal Medicine* **121**: 1–5.

31. Greenman RL, Schein RMH, Martin MA *et al.* (1991) A controlled clinical trial of E5 murine monoclonal IgM antibody to endotoxin in the treatment of Gram-negative sepsis. *Journal of the American Medical Association* **226**: 1097–1102.

32. Giroir BP, Quint PA, Barton P *et al.* (1997) Preliminary evaluation of recombinant amino-terminal fragment of human bactericidal/permeability-increasing protein in children with severe meningococcal sepsis. *Lancet* **350**: 1439–1443.

33. Pinsky MR, Vincent JL, Deviere J *et al.* (1993) Serum cytokine levels in human septic shock: relation to multiple-systems organ failure and mortality. *Chest* **103**: 565–575.

34. Stephens KE, Ishizaka A, Larrick JW *et al.* (1998) Tumor necrosis factor causes increased pulmonary permeability and edema. *American Review of Respiratory Diseases* **137**: 1364–1370.

35. Van der Poll T, Van Deventer SJ, ten Cate H *et al.* (1994) Tumor necrosis factor is involved in the appearance of interleukin-1 receptor antagonist in endotoxemia. *Journal of Infectious Diseases* **169**: 665–667.

36. Opal SM, Cross AS, Kelly NM *et al.* (1990) Efficacy of a monoclonal antibody directed against tumor necrosis factor in protecting neutropenic rats from lethal infection with *Pseudomonas aeruginosa. Journal of Infectious Diseases* **161**: 1148–1152.

37. Cohen J, Carlet J, INTERSEPT Study Group (1996) INTERSEPT: an international, multicenter, placebo-controlled trial of monoclonal antibody to human tumor necrosis factor – in patients with sepsis. *Critical Care Medicine* **24**: 1431–1440.

38. Waage A, Espevik T (1998) Interleukin-1 potentiates the lethal effect of tumor necrosis factor α/cachecin in mice. *Journal of Experimental Medicine* **167**: 1987–1992.

39. Hosenpud JD (1993) The effects of interleukin 1 on myocardial function and metabolism. *Clinical Immunology and Immunopathology* **68**: 175–180.

40. Fischer E, Marano MA, Van Zee KJ *et al.* (1992) Interleukin-1 receptor blockade improves survival and hemodynamic performance in *Escherichia coli* septic shock, but fails to alter host responses to sublethal endotoxemia. *Journal of Clinical Investigation* **89**: 1551–1557.

41. Fischer CJ, Slotman GJ, Opal SM *et al.* (1994) Initial evaluation of human recombinant interleukin-1 receptor antagonist in the treatment of sepsis syndrome: a randomized, open-label, placebo-controlled multicenter trial. *Critical Care Medicine* **22**: 12–21.

42. Opal SM, Fischer CJ Jr., Dhainaut JF *et al.* (1997) Confirmatory interleukin-1 receptor antagonist trial in severe sepsis: a phase III, randomized, double-blind, placebo-controlled, multicenter trial. *Critical Care Medicine* **25**: 1115–1124.

43. Chang SW, Feddersen CO, Henson PM *et al.* Platelet-activating factor mediates hemodynamic changes and lung injury in endotoxin-treated rats. *Journal of Clinical Investigation* **79**: 1498–1509.

44. Myers AK, Robey JW (1990) Relationships between tumour necrosis factors, eicosanoids and platelet-activating factor as mediators of endotoxin-induced shock in mice. *British Journal of Pharmacology* **99**: 499–502.

45. Dhainaut JF, Tenaillon A, Le Tulzo Y *et al.* (1994) Platelet activating receptor antagonist BN52021 in the treatment of severe sepsis: a randomized, double-blind, placebo-controlled, multicenter clinical trial. BN 52021 Sepsis Study Group. *Critical Care Medicine* **22**: 1720–1728.

46. Neuhof H (1991) Actions and interactions of mediators systems and mediators in the pathogenesis of ARDS and multiorgan failure. *Acta Anaesthesiologica Scandinavica* **35**: 7–14.

47. Bernard GR, Wheeler AP, Arons M *et al.* (1997) A trial of antioxidants *N*-acetyl cysteine and procysteine in ARDS. *Chest* **112**: 164–172.

48. Finkel MS, Oddis CV, Jacob TD *et al.* (1997) Negative inotropic effects of cytokines on the heart mediated by nitric oxide. *Science* **257**: 378–389.

49. Nguyen T, Brunson D, Crespi CL *et al.* (1992) DNA damage and mutation in human cells exposed to nitric oxide *in vitro. Proceedings of the National Academy of Sciences of the USA* **89**: 3030–3034.

50. Petros A, Lamb G, Leone A *et al.* (1994) Effects of a nitric oxide synthase inhibitor in humans with septic shock. *Cardiovascular Research* **28**: 34–39.

51. Zhang H, Rogiers P, Preiser JC *et al.* (1995) Effects of methylene blue on oxygen availability and regional blood flow during endotoxic shock. *Critical Care Medicine* **23**: 1711–1721.

52. Preiser JC, Lejeune P, Roman A *et al.* (1995) Methylene blue administration in septic shock: a clinical trial. *Critical Care Medicine* **23**: 259–264.

53. Rees DD, Cellek S, Palmer RM et al. (1990) Dexamethasone prevents the induction by endotoxin of a nitric oxide synthase and the associated effects on vascular tone: an insight into endotoxin shock. *Biochemical and Biophysical Research Communications* **173**: 541–547.

54. The Veterans Administration Systemic Sepsis Cooperative Study Group (1987) Effect of high-dose glucocorticoid therapy on mortality in patients with clinical signs of systemic sepsis. *New England Journal of Medicine* **317**: 659–665.

55. Bernard GR, Luce JM, Sprung CL et al. (1987) High-dose corticosteroids in patients with the adult respiratory distress syndrome. *New England Journal of Medicine* **317**: 1565–1570.

56. Bollaert PE, Charpentier C, Levy B et al. (1998) Reversal of late septic shock with supraphysiologic doses of hydrocortisone. *Critical Care Medicine* **26**: 645–650.

57. Eichacker PQ, Waisman Y, Natanson C et al. (1994) Cardiopulmonary effects of granulocyte colony stimulating factor in a canine model of bacterial sepsis. *Journal of Applied Physiology* **77**: 2366–2373.

58. Weiss M, Gross-Weege W, Schneider M et al. (1995) Enhancement of neutrophil function by *in vivo* filgrastim treatment for prophylaxis of sepsis in surgical intensive care patients. *Journal of Critical Care* **10**: 21–26.

Section 2

System-Based Infection

7 Respiratory infections

Infections of the respiratory tract are amongst the most common and the most serious in the intensive care unit (ICU). Respiratory tract infections may be classified into upper and lower, but the latter are more common in the severely ill adult patient. Serious infections of the upper respiratory tract are commoner in childhood but those included here, although relatively unusual, may be life-threatening. It is important to obtain a microbiological diagnosis to confirm the aetiology, indicate the likely prognosis and guide specific antibiotic therapy.

UPPER RESPIRATORY INFECTIONS

Epiglottitis

This is a relatively uncommon condition in adults. It is characterized by swelling and oedema of the epiglottis and the surrounding tissue structures, and the clinical presentation in adults is usually less acute than during childhood. Nonetheless, it may present requiring securement of the airway and then immediate ICU admission.

Presentation

Sudden partial or complete obstruction of the airways with fever and respiratory distress are common. There may be a recent history of sore throat, hoarseness and possibly dysphagia, and rapid deterioration with loss of consciousness and cardiorespiratory arrest may occur in a matter of minutes.

Diagnosis

The above together with a red, inflamed epiglottis (examination should occur only after securing the airway) is suggestive of the diagnosis. Diphtheria, angioneurotic oedema, a peritonsillar abscess and large airways obstruction caused by a foreign body are amongst the differential diagnoses. Blood cultures and a swab obtained from the epiglottis, after the airway has been secured, will help confirm a microbiological diagnosis. Severe epiglottitis in the adult may be viral in origin or caused by bacteria such as *Streptococcus pneumoniae* or *Haemophilus influenzae*.

Management

It is essential to secure the airway immediately by means of an endotracheal or nasotracheal tube. An intravenous cephalosporin such as cefuroxime, 1.5 g 8-hourly, or cefotaxime, 1–2 g 8-hourly, should be administered for 7–10 days;

the increasing incidence of β-lactamase-producing isolates of *H. influenzae* and penicillin-resistant *S. pneumoniae* precludes the use of ampicillin or benzylpenicillin as blind initial therapy.

Diphtheria

Humans are the only known source of *Corynebacterium diphtheriae*, a pleomorphic Gram-positive bacillus, which may be isolated from the respiratory tract and skin. Phages mediate the production of an exotoxin which causes local inflammation and inhibits protein synthesis in human cells, especially the heart (causing myocarditis), nervous system (causing demyelination) and kidney (causing tubular necrosis). Vaccination with a toxoid vaccine at 2, 3 and 4 months of age, usually administered with tetanus, whooping cough, polio and *H. influenzae* type b vaccines, has largely eradicated this infection in most developed countries. In recent years there has been an increase in the incidence of infection in the former Soviet bloc countries due to a fall-off in the vaccination rate, and partial or progressive waning of immune protection in adults in the absence of recommended booster vaccines elsewhere necessitates continued awareness and appropriate investigation of this uncommon but serious infection[1].

Presentation

Fever, malaise, dysphagia and a severe sore throat should prompt consideration of diphtheria in the differential diagnosis. The presence of a white and glistening membrane on both tonsils, the uvula and soft palate is characteristic (Plate 5). Lymphadenopathy with severe swelling and oedema (bullneck), and tracheitis and bronchitis leading to respiratory distress, may also occur. Complications include local paralysis of the palate and larynx, peripheral neuritis and myocarditis.

Diagnosis

Diphtheria should be considered as a possible diagnosis in any patient with a severe sore throat, especially if accompanied by a membrane on examination,

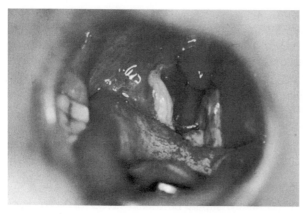

Plate 5 Tonsillar membrane characteristic of diphtheria. (Courtesy of Dr I. Zamiri; published in Emond RTD *et al.* (1995) *Colour Atlas of Infectious Diseases*, 3rd edit. Mosby-Wolfe: London.)

who has not been vaccinated, or whose vaccination status is unknown, or who has recently travelled or resided in an area where vaccination rates are low. The differential diagnosis will also include severe streptococcal pharyngitis, infectious mononucleosis, Vincent's angina and epiglottitis (see above). Confirmation of the diagnosis is made by isolating the bacterium from the throat but it is important that the microbiology laboratory be informed of the possible diagnosis in advance, as culture for *C. diphtheriae* from throat swabs is no longer routine in many laboratories. Selective media such as tellurite or Tinsdale agar are required to inhibit the growth of normal throat commensals and thereby facilitate the isolation of *C. diphtheriae*. The reference laboratory should also confirm that the isolate is toxin positive by the Elek test (an *in vitro* antibody–antigen test) or increasingly by the polymerase chain reaction (PCR), as non-toxin-producing strains are less virulent and contacts of the patient do not then require follow-up.

Management

Patients with severe infection may require intubation and ventilation. Antibiotics reduce the severity of infection, render patients less infectious and inhibit the production of toxin with its consequent effects. The recommended antibiotic treatment is erythromycin, i.v., 500 mg 6-hourly, or benzylpenicillin, i.v., 1.8 g 6-hourly. Diphtheria antitoxin, e.g. 40 000–100 000 units, should be given intramuscularly or intravenously in severe infection, i.e. patients with extensive membrane or severe oedema[2]. Patients with diphtheria should be isolated, preferably in a negatively ventilated room, until culture negative for *C. diphtheriae* to prevent spread to other patients. Diphtheria is notifiable in the UK and most other countries and it is essential that close contacts of the patient within the previous 7 days are screened for the bacterium and given antibiotics. Therefore close collaboration between intensivists, medical microbiologists and public health physicians is essential in the successful management of this condition.

Sinusitis

This is not often an indication *per se* for admission to the ICU, but should be considered in the differential diagnosis of any ICU patient with a temperature for which there is no obvious source. Furthermore, sinus infection may be a continuing source of infection in patients with ventilator-associated pneumonia refractory to antibiotic treatment. It is increasingly recognized as a cause of ICU-acquired pneumonia even in non-ventilated but intubated patients. Risk factors for sinusitis in the ICU patient include craniofacial injury, prolonged nasogastric or nasotracheal intubation and steroids[3]. A diagnosis may be confirmed by standard sinus radiography or computed tomography (CT) or magnetic resonance imaging (MRI), which may reveal total opacification or an air fluid level (Figure 7.1). Sinus puncture and culture is recommended to guide appropriate antimicrobial therapy, and any nasal tubes should be removed if at all possible. Gram-negative bacilli predominate as pathogens but infection is often polymicrobial. Many studies have confirmed the simultaneous colonization of the sinuses and the tracheobronchial tree, with a strong association between

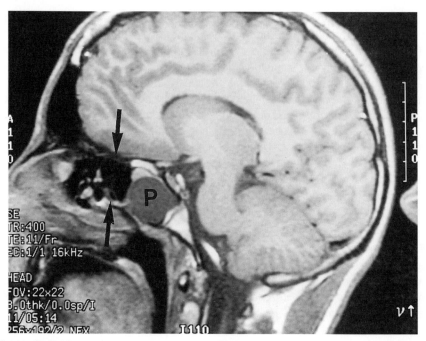

Figure 7.1 Magnetic resonance imaging (MRI) scan demonstrating a pyocele (P) completely filling the sphenoid sinus. Normal sinuses containing air should be black as in the ethmoidal air cells (arrows).

nosocomial sinusitis and pneumonia; occasionally sinus drainage is required to treat pneumonia effectively[3].

LOWER RESPIRATORY INFECTIONS

Lower respiratory tract infection is a somewhat vague term used in the ICU. 'Pneumonia' implies inflammation and infection of the alveolar spaces, i.e. parenchymal involvement, but it is difficult to distinguish clinically from airways infection. 'Pneumonitis', i.e. inflammation of the interalveolar spaces, is also sometimes used. In practice, these distinctions are less important unless there is confirmation of the diagnosis by histology following lung biopsy and treatment has to be altered, but different terminologies for the same clinical condition sometimes lead to confusion. A clear distinction should be made, however, between lower respiratory tract infection in the patient with an intact immune system and infection in the patient who is immunocompromised, as the approach to investigation and management differs (see below and also Chapter 12).

Community-acquired pneumonia

Most patients with community-acquired pneumonia do not require admission to hospital and an even smaller proportion require ICU care. Community-acquired pneumonia is, however, a common cause of admission to the ICU, accounting for as many as 10% of all admissions to medical ICUs[4].

Presentation

Common clinical features are cough, productive sputum (may be absent in atypical pneumonia), chest pain, high fever and consolidation on examination and chest X-ray. Specific features of patients with community-acquired infection requiring ICU care include[4]:

1. Respiratory rate of over 30 min^{-1}
2. Pao_2 of less than 8 kPa
3. Serum urea concentration over 7 mmol l^{-1}
4. Lymphopenia
5. Alteration in mental status

Stratification of patients according to underlying disease, physical features on admission to hospital and abnormal laboratory findings can be used to guide management and predict prognosis, and those with the greatest number of risk factors are more likely to need admission to the ICU[5]. Cavitation on chest X-ray, described in the past as a common feature of staphylococcal pneumonia, is now unusual due to the earlier administration of antibiotics, and the radiological features of pneumonia may vary from non-specific findings to frank consolidation, pleural effusion and even empyema. Viral pneumonia is relatively rare, except during influenza outbreaks, but can nonetheless be severe; varicella pneumonia, characterized by cough and dyspnoea occurring approximately 6 days after the onset of rash, may be accompanied by a degree of hypoxia, often not clinically very apparent[6, 7].

Diagnosis

In addition to a full clinical assessment (e.g. contact with birds may suggest psittacosis, travel abroad from the UK may suggest legionellosis), a full blood count, urea and electrolytes, blood gases and chest X-ray (Figure 7.2), efforts should be made to confirm a microbiological diagnosis to guide specific antimicrobial therapy (Table 7.1) Where at all possible, specimens obtained at bronchoscopy, i.e. bronchoalveolar lavage (BAL) or protected brush specimens (PBS), should be submitted for microbiological investigation in preference to sputa, especially in very ill patients, to diagnose unusual causes of infection or to exclude non-infective pathology (Figure 7.3).

Many patients may be admitted to the ICU after receiving one or more antibiotics without having had a full investigation. Blood should be cultured from most patients with community-acquired pneumonia[8]. For example, S. pneumoniae isolated from blood cultures may confirm the aetiology but this finding also indicates a poorer prognosis than when the organism is isolated from the respiratory tract alone. Additional laboratory investigations, such as Legionella antigen detection in respiratory specimens and urine, should be

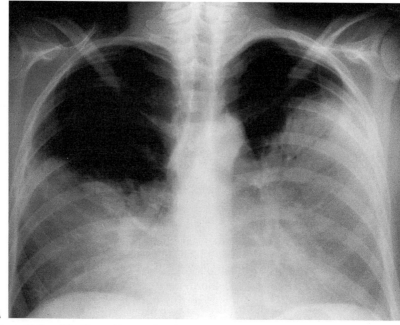

A

Figure 7.2 (A) Chest X-ray of pneumococcal pneumonia with involvement of both the middle and lower lung fields.

considered in patients who may have so-called atypical pneumonia, e.g. the returned traveller with a dry cough and flu-like symptoms (Table 7.1). In practice, severe community-acquired pneumonia requiring admission to the ICU caused by typical and atypical agents may be clinically and radiologically indistinguishable. Although the pneumococcus is the commonest cause of community-acquired pneumonia, there is now greater recognition of other pathogens such as *Chlamydia pneumoniae* and these are likely to be increasingly important with the advent of improved diagnostic techniques (see Chapter 4). For example, it is believed that *C. pneumoniae* may be responsible for up to 20% of cases of community-acquired pneumonia and in the elderly it is responsible for severe disease[9].

Treatment

Initial blind treatment must cover *S. pneumoniae*, which is responsible for about 60–70% of cases, and atypical organisms especially when infection is severe. A second- or third-generation cephalosporin, e.g. cefuroxime, i.v., 1.5 g 8-hourly, or cefotaxime, i.v., 2 g 8-hourly (especially if altered immune status such as cirrhosis), will cover both *H. influenzae*, penicillin-sensitive and penicillin-resistant *S. pneumoniae* (where prevalent), but benzylpenicillin (i.v., 1.8 g 6-hourly) should be substituted if a sensitive strain of *S. pneumoniae* is isolated. Erythromycin, i.v., 500 mg 6-hourly, covers *Legionella* and *Mycoplasma* infection, and has reasonable activity against *Chlamydia*. Modifications to the above may be

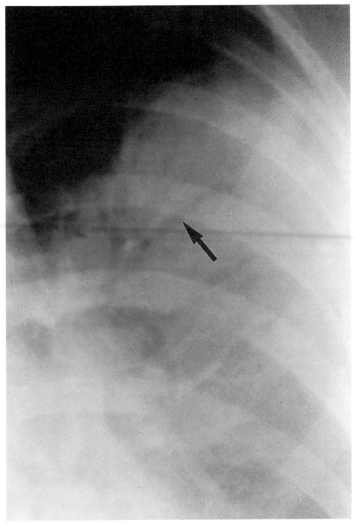

Figure 7.2 (B) Detail of the left midzone shows air bronchogram (arrow).

required following the results of culture and sensitivities of the locally prevalent pathogen, especially if resistant bacteria are responsible for infection. Five to ten days of antibiotics should be adequate for common bacterial pneumonia, 10–14 days is required for infections caused by *Mycoplasma pneumoniae* or *C. pneumoniae* and 14–21 days is recommended for legionnaires' disease[8].

Acute exacerbation of chronic obstructive pulmonary disease (COPD)

Only a small proportion of patients with COPD require ICU care and a decision to ventilate will depend on whether this is likely to benefit the individual patient

Table 7.1 Microbiological investigations of patients admitted to the ICU with community-acquired pneumonia.

Aetiology	Investigations
Typical S. pneumoniae H. influenzae Staphylococcus aureus	Respiratory samples for microscopy and culture[a] Two sets of blood cultures, urine and pleural fluid for pneumococcal antigen
Atypical Legionella spp.	Respiratory samples for specialist culture[a], paired serum samples[b], urine and respiratory samples for antigen detection.
Mycoplasma pneumoniae Chlamydia psittaci C. pneumoniae	Paired serum samples[b], antigen detection in respiratory samples
Influenza virus and adenoviruses	Paired serum samples[b], throat and lower respiratory samples for antigen detection and viral culture

[a] Bronchoscopy samples (e.g. bronchoalveolar lavage or protected brush specimens) should be obtained where possible and discussed with the microbiology laboratory to ensure appropriate processing.
[b] 5–10 ml of blood 7–10 days apart to document a fourfold rise in antibody titre or a single high titre.

Pneumonia suspected if:
Two temperature spikes >38.5°C over a 24-hour period
White cell count >12 000 or <4 000 x 10^9L^{-1}

Diagnosis confirmed if three of the following present
Purulent sputum or tracheal aspirate
New infiltrates on chest X-ray
An increase of 0.15 in FIo_2 to maintain equivalent oxygenation
Positive culture from BAL or PBS
NB Bronchopneumonia predominates on the right;
bronchoscopy may be required to confirm
the aetiology of left lung infiltrates.
Microscopy of BAL or PBS specimens may provide
a presumptive diagnosis if organisms,
especially if intracellular, are seen

Figure 7.3 Approach to confirming a diagnosis of ICU-acquired pneumonia.

in the short and long term. Infection is not always the cause of acute exacerbations (changes in air quality are probably underestimated) but where infection is responsible viruses are probably at least as common as bacteria but do not warrant the routine use of antibacterial agents.

Presentation
Respiratory failure in a patient with underlying chronic bronchitis and emphysema with or without fever or purulent sputum is characteristic. In patients with severe emphysema and lower respiratory tract infection, there may be few if any opacities seen on the chest X-ray due to distorted and expanded alveolar spaces leading to minimal lung tissue, compared with consolidation characteristic of pneumonia (Figure 7.2)

Diagnosis
Sputum or preferably BAL or PBS (especially if the patient is very ill) should be obtained. Blood cultures are generally indicated if there is fever or other evidence of systemic infection.

Management
Antibacterial treatment is not indicated if the patient is apyrexial, the sputum is non-purulent and the chest X-ray is normal. Non-encapsulated H. influenzae, S. pneumoniae and Moraxella (formerly known as Branhamella) catarrhalis are the commonest causes of acute exacerbation and, although antibiotics may not eradicate airways carriage of these bacteria, antibiotic therapy results in a statistically significant acceleration of recovery, especially in patients with frequent or recurrent infection[10]. Cefuroxime, i.v., 1.5 g 8-hourly, or co-amoxiclav, i.v., 1.2 g 8-hourly, is recommended depending upon local patterns of resistance.

Ventilator-associated pneumonia
Ventilator-associated pneumonia occurs at least 48–72 hours after intubation. The aetiology and pathogenesis is different in many respects to pneumonia acquired in the community but there is some overlap between nosocomial pneumonia, i.e. infection acquired in any area of the hospital, and that acquired in the ICU. Organisms colonizing the oropharynx and stomach, i.e. endogenous organisms, may track along the endotracheal tube and subsequently cause pneumonia; bacteria from respiratory devices, from other equipment and from other patients, i.e. exogenous organisms, are a less frequent source[11]. Enterobacteriaceae such as Escherichia coli, Enterobacter cloacae and Serratia marcescens, Pseudomonas aeruginosa, Acinetobacter spp. and S. aureus are the major causes.

Large-scale aspiration in the ICU patient is unusual but when it occurs it is usually clinically and radiologically apparent. Low-grade aspiration does not always warrant antibiotic treatment unless there is clinical, radiological or microbiological evidence of infection. Overall, the rate of ventilator-associated pneumonia is 14.8 cases per 1000 ventilator days or 3% per day during the first week of mechanical ventilation, the risk factors being[12]:

1. Burns as an admission diagnosis
2. Trauma
3. Central nervous system disease
4. Respiratory or cardiovascular disease
5. Ventilation during the previous 24 hours
6. Witnessed aspiration and paralysing agents

There is an inverse relationship between ventilator-associated pneumonia and antibiotic use which confirms recent reviews on the efficacy of selective decontamination of the digestive tract (SDD) (see Chapters 3 and 10).

Presentation
There are no distinctive characteristics that facilitate an easy diagnosis and chest X-ray findings are often non-specific. Fever, increasing purulent secretions, deteriorating blood gases, a low or high peripheral white cell count (i.e. <3 or >15 × 10^9 l^{-1}) and new shadows on a chest X-ray are all features consistent with the diagnosis, but some or all of these findings may also be seen in patients with the acute respiratory distress syndrome (ARDS), patients following severe chest trauma with haemorrhage, or patients with cardiac failure.

Diagnosis
Following intubation, the lower airways become colonized by potential pathogens and consequently culture of sputum or tracheal aspirates is not specific enough. Confirmation of the diagnosis is problematic, invasive techniques are either not always available or cost effective and there have been no good studies to indicate the impact of diagnostic approaches on outcome[13]. Nonetheless, non-quantitative analysis of endotracheal aspirates overestimates the diagnosis of ventilator-associated pnuemonia as it includes tracheobronchial colonization or non-infectious processes. Whilst BAL and PBS are time consuming and not always available, semi-quantitation of endotracheal culture results provides a realistic alternative and it is now strongly recommended. With this kind of approach, antibiotics should not be given to patients without pathogenic micro-organisms[14]. Microscopy of BAL or PBS specimens may assist in choosing initial antibiotic therapy and quantitation of culture results is recommended in patients with the features described above; if at all clinically possible, anti-biotics should be discontinued for 48 hours beforehand[11]. A protocol for the use of BAL or PBS in the ICU is described in Figure 7.3 and the unit should have a procedure in place for decontamination of the bronchoscope after use.

Non-bronchoscopic lavage with quantitation of culture results, which requires less expertise and may be more feasible in smaller ICUs, is a useful alternative especially where there are no specific indications for bronchoscopy, such as obtaining lung tissue to exclude malignancy[15]. Occasionally the processing of such specimens for other pathogens such as legionnaires' disease (Table 7.1) is required depending upon the possible source and clinical circumstances. Two sets of blood cultures are also mandatory to confirm bacteraemic pneumonia, which has a poorer prognosis, and which may necessitate more than one antibiotic for a successful outcome. Confirming a microbiological diagnosis is important as the outcome is partly determined by the aetiology; patients with pneumonia due to methicillin-resistant *S. aureus* (MRSA) and non-fermenting Gram-negative bacilli such as *P. aeruginosa* and *Acinetobacter* spp. have a poorer prognosis[16].

Management

Depending upon local antimicrobial sensitivity patterns, initial empirical therapy should cover Gram-negative bacilli (including *P. aeruginosa*) and *S. aureus* and may be influenced by whether infection is early or late onset, and whether the patient has recently been on antibiotics. Opinion continues to be divided on the benefits of combination treatment compared with monotherapy; an expanded spectrum of activity, a reduced likelihood of resistance emerging and potential synergy are arguments in favour of combination therapy.

An aminoglycoside administered in sufficiently high dosage to achieve good serum and tissue levels with a β-lactam agent (e.g. a cephalosporin with antipseudomonal activity) is a commonly recommended approach[17]. In severe or bacteraemic pneumonia, an aminoglycoside (e.g. gentamicin, i.v., $5\,mg\,kg^{-1}$ daily in one dose) in combination with ciprofloxacin (i.v., 400 mg 12-hourly), ceftazidime (i.v., 2 g 8-hourly), or tazobactam/piperacillin (i.v., 4.5 g 8-hourly) is advised. Following the results of sensitivity tests, the initial regimen may subsequently be changed. In ICUs where MRSA is endemic, vancomycin (i.v., 1 g 12-hourly) or teicoplanin (400 mg 12-hourly for three doses followed by 400 mg daily) should also be considered as part of the initial regimen. Serum aminoglycoside (pre-dose) or vancomycin (pre- and post-dose samples) assays are required in all patients receiving these agents for 48 hours or longer to confirm therapeutic levels are achieved and to detect early toxic side-effects. Seven to ten days' antibiotic treatment should usually be adequate but the duration of treatment will be influenced by the needs of the individual patient, the aetiology (e.g. longer courses are required for *Pseudomonas* infection) and the initial response to treatment. Repeat BAL or PBS is indicated where there is a poor response to therapy, to exclude the emergence of resistant pathogens whilst on therapy or to detect an additional pathogen which was not present or isolated initially.

Patients who develop empyema or a lung abscess will usually require aspiration and drainage either under radiological guidance (e.g. ultrasonography) or at operation. Fresh samples of pus or drainage fluid should be sent for culture to guide changes in antimicrobial therapy; samples taken from chest drains are less useful. Pus or fluid that has collected in drainage bags is unreliable as overgrowth at room temperature of non-significant bacteria may occur.

97

Pulmonary tuberculosis

Pulmonary tuberculosis (TB) is uncommon in most ICUs in developed countries but this infection remains important because of the emergence of multi-drug-resistant strains in the HIV population, the increasing mobility amongst immigrants and the socially deprived, who are at particular risk, and because 'open' TB is potentially very infectious, especially in a clinical area with severely ill patients such as the ICU. Multi-drug-resistant TB remains a challenge in terms of determining the most appropriate chemotherapeutic regimen and preventing spread to other patients and health care workers. A recent survey in the UK revealed an overall incidence of isoniazid resistance of 6%, and multi-drug resistance of 2%, but with almost three times those levels in HIV-positive patients[18].

Presentation

TB should be considered in any ICU patient with a previous history of infection, in patients with recent symptoms compatible with TB (e.g. persistent cough, weight loss, haemoptysis), in all patients in at-risk groups (e.g. immigrants, HIV-positive individuals, alcoholics) presenting with respiratory infection, and in any patient with characteristic chest X-ray findings such as upper lobe fibrosis and cavitation (Figure 7.4) and possibly in any patient with persistent respiratory infection for which no cause has been identified.

Diagnosis

In addition to chest X-ray, up to three sputa or tracheal aspirates should be sent for Ziehl–Neelsen or auramine staining and TB culture. BAL or PBS specimens should be obtained if these specimens are negative or difficult to obtain. However, BAL, PBS or other bronchoscopic specimens that are microscopy positive for TB do not represent 'open' TB unless sputum or tracheal aspirates are also positive. There is less of a role for skin testing in the ICU because these patients are somewhat immunocompromised and false-negative results are possible.

Management

Patients with TB should preferably be managed by a respiratory or an infectious disease physician in conjunction with the intensivist to monitor therapy, manage side-effects and ensure continuation of treatment after discharge from the ICU. A regimen consisting of isoniazid, rifampicin, ethambutol and pyrazinamide given for 2 months, followed by isoniazid and rifampicin for 4 months, is recommended for patients with fully susceptible organisms and for patients who adhere to treatment[19, 20]. TB is notifiable and management must also consider spread to other patients and health care personnel following the diagnosis of 'open' tuberculosis.

Pneumonia in the immunocompromised patient

As advances continue to be made in the treatment of malignancy and the antiviral chemotherapy of AIDS, increasing numbers of immunocompromised

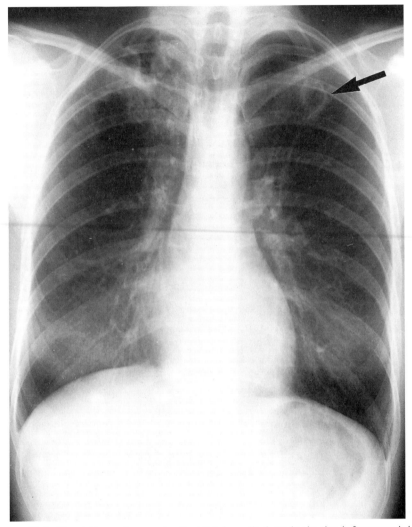

Figure 7.4 Chest X-ray demonstrating thick-walled cavity in the left upper lobe (arrow) with additional cavities and fibrotic changes in the right apex characteristic of TB.

patients are likely to be admitted to the ICU for ventilation or organ support. Other immunocompromised patients who may require ICU care include patients with severe congenital immunodeficiency, patients with neutropenia due to antitumour chemotherapy or an underlying haematological malignancy, patients following bone marrow or solid organ transplantation, and patients on high-dose corticosteroids or other immunosuppressive agents such as cyclosporin. Although the majority of patients requiring admission to the ICU are severely ill and are vulnerable to infection with conventional pathogens such as *P. aeruginosa* discussed above, immunocompromised patients are vulnerable to a range of other opportunist pathogens. Furthermore, pneumonia in such patients may be part of a systemic infection affecting other organs, e.g. cytomegalovirus infection causing pneumonia, hepatitis and colitis, which may influence treatment. HIV-positive patients are also at a higher risk of contracting respiratory tract infection caused by *C. pneumoniae* and this may occur with other pathogens[9]. For further details of other infections, see Chapter 12.

Presentation

Increasing respiratory distress leading to respiratory failure in any category of patient listed above should be attributable to infection until proven otherwise and merits full investigation. Conventional symptoms of lower respiratory tract infection (e.g. purulent sputum) and clinical or radiological signs (e.g. fever, consolidation) may be absent.

Diagnosis

The category of patient and the nature of the immunosuppression may give some clue to the likely microbiological aetiology. For example, during the initial period following bone marrow transplantation when patients are likely to be neutropenic, common Gram-positive and Gram-negative bacteria as well as *Aspergillus* spp. should be considered. Later, i.e. from 3 months onwards, cytomegalovirus and *Pneumocystis carinii* become more common. Unless otherwise contraindicated, such as during severe thrombocytopenia, bronchoscopy is strongly recommended to obtain good-quality specimens, and to visualize the bronchial tree. There is now a wide range of potential laboratory investigations available[21], some of which are confined to larger centres or reference laboratories, and the diagnosis of some of the more common pathogens in these patients is outlined in Table 7.2. Lung biopsy is now rarely carried out following the more widespread availability of bronchoscopy and other techniques to obtain appropriate respiratory specimens. Even in immunocompromised patients, the results of open lung biopsy rarely lead to clinical benefit although they may result in a change of therapy[22]. Fungal pneumonia, only truly confirmed by histological evidence of tissue invasion (Plate 6), is now rarely diagnosed by open lung biopsy due to the risks of such a procedure in a severely ill patient. However, this procedure may be indicated to exclude non-infective conditions such as malignancy, which will subsequently influence the overall management of the patient.

Treatment

This will depend on the specific aetiology and details of this are provided in Chapter 12. Empirical therapy before the results of investigations, however, may have to include broad-spectrum antibacterial cover, including cover against *P. aeruginosa* (e.g. a third-generation cephalosporin such as ceftazidime, i.v., 2 g

Table 7.2 Laboratory diagnosis of some common respiratory pathogens in immunocompromised patients.

Infection	Laboratory diagnosis
Pneumocystis carinii	Antigen detection using fluorescent microscopy, PCR[a]
Aspergillus spp.	Routine and calcofluor fluorescent microscopy, fungal culture, PCR[a]
Cytomegalovirus	Antigen detection using fluorescent microscopy, culture with early fluorescent antigen detection, PCR[a]
Mycobacterium tuberculosis and other species	Ziehl–Neelsen stain, culture, PCR[a]

[a] PCR is still in the developmental stage and available in some centres but is likely to become routine in the near future.

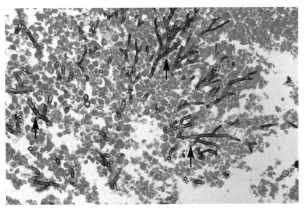

Plate 6 Histological section of lung tissue (Grocot stain) demonstrating hyphae (arrows) indicative of invasive aspergillosis.

8-hourly, and an aminoglycoside, i.v., 5 mg kg^{-1} once daily), anti-*Pneumocystis* therapy (e.g. high-dose co-trimoxazole, 120 mg kg^{-1} day^{-1} divided into three to four doses) and an antifungal agent such as amphotericin B. Therapy of *Pneumocystis* infection should initially be administered intravenously and serum levels of co-trimoxazole may need to be determined to minimize the incidence of side-effects[23]. It is important to remember that a poor response to treatment may be due to other infections or extrapulmonary *Pneumocystis* infection, and the radiological appearances may lag behind clinical improvement[23]. Management of infection in this complex group of patients should involve the intensivist, haematologist/oncologist, microbiologist, infectious disease physician and respiratory physician.

Key points

- Respiratory infections, especially those of the lower tract, are a major cause of mortality and morbidity in the ICU.
- Diphtheria should be considered in any patient with a severe sore throat who has not been vaccinated, or who has recently been working or living in a country with low vaccination rates.
- *S. pneumoniae* is responsible for over 60% of cases of community-acquired pneumonia.
- BAL or PSB or equivalent should be used to confirm the diagnosis of ventilator-associated pneumonia and to guide antimicrobial chemotherapy.
- The diagnosis and management of respiratory infection in immunosuppressed patients requires specialist laboratory investigations and liaison with the relevant specialties.

REFERENCES

1. Rey M (1996) Resurgence of diphtheria in Europe. *Clinical Microbiology and Infection* **2**: 71–73.
2. Department of Health (1996) *Immunization Against Infectious Diseases*. Her Majesty's Stationary Office, London.
3. Bert F, Lambert-Zechovsky N (1996) Sinusitis in mechanically ventilated patients and its role in the pathogenesis of nosocomial pneumonia. *European Journal of Clinical Microbiology and Infectious Diseases* **15**: 533–544.
4. British Thoracic Society Research Committee and Public Health Laboratory Service (1992) The aetiology, management and outcome of severe community-acquired pneumonia on the intensive care unit. *Respiratory Medicine* **86**: 7–13.
5. Fine MJ, Auble TE, Yealy DM et al. (1997) A prediction rule to identify low-risk patients with community-acquired pneumonia. *New England Journal of Medicine* **336**: 243–250.
6. Arvin AM (1996) Varicella-zoster virus. *Clinical Microbiology Reviews* **9**: 361–381.
7. Cohen JI, Brunell PA, Straus SE et al. (1999) Recent advances in varicella-zoster infection. *New England Journal of Medicine* **130**: 922–932.
8. Bartlett G, Mundy LM (1995) Community-acquired pneumonia. *New England Journal of Medicine* **333**: 1618–1624.
9. Blasi F, Tarsia P, Arosio C et al. (1998) Epidemiology of *Chlamydia pneumoniae*. *Clinical Microbiology and Infection* **4**: 4S1–4S6.
10. Murphy TF, Sethi S (1992) Bacterial infection in chronic obstructive pulmonary disease. *American Review of Respiratory Disease* **146**: 1067–1083.
11. Francioli P, Chastre J, Langer M et al. (1997) Ventilator-associated pneumonia – understanding epidemiology and pathogenesis to guide prevention and empiric therapy. *Clinical Microbiology and Infection* **3**: S61–S76.
12. Cook DJ, Walter SD, Cook RJ et al. (1998) Incidence of risk factors for ventilator-associated pneumonia in critically ill patients. *Annals of Internal Medicine* **129**: 433–440.

13. Flanagan PG (1999) Diagnosis of ventilator-associated pneumonia. *Journal of Hospital Infection* **41**: 87–99.
14. Pittet D, Harbarth S (1998) What techniques for diagnosis of ventilator-associated pneumonia? *Lancet* **352**: 83–84.
15. Humphreys H, Winter R, Baker M *et al.* (1996) Comparison of bronchoalveolar lavage and catheter lavage to confirm ventilator-associated lower respiratory tract infection. *Journal of Medical Microbiology* **45**: 226–231.
16. Rello J, Valles J (1998) Mortality as an outcome in hospital-acquired pneumonia. *Infection Control and Hospital Epidemiology* **19**: 795–797.
17. Brown EM (1997) Empirical antimicrobial therapy of mechanically ventilated patients with nosocomial pneumonia. *Journal of Antimicrobial Chemotherapy* **40**: 463–468.
18. Irish C, Herbert J, Bennett D *et al.* (1999) Database study of antibiotic-resistant tuberculosis in the United Kingdom, 1994–6. *British Medical Journal* **318**: 497–498.
19. American Thoracic Society (1994) Treatment of tuberculosis and tuberculosis infection in adults and children. *American Journal of Respiratory and Critical Care Medicine* **149**: 1359–1374.
20. Joint Tuberculosis Committee of the British Thoracic Society (1998) Chemotherapy and management of tuberculosis in the United Kingdom: recommendations 1998. *Thorax* **53**: 536–548.
21. Shelhamer JH, Gill VJ, Quinn TC *et al.* (1996) The laboratory evaluation of opportunistic pulmonary infections. *Annals of Internal Medicine* **124**: 585–599.
22. Lode H, Schaberg T, Raffenberg M *et al.* (1993) Diagnostic problems in lower respiratory tract infections. *Journal of Antimicrobial Chemotherapy* **32** (Suppl A): 29–37.
23. Fishman JA (1998) Treatment of infection due to *Pneumocystis carinii*. *Antimicrobial Agents and Chemotherapy* **42**: 1309–1314.

8 Systemic infections

INTRODUCTION

Early mortality in critically ill patients has fallen with improvements in resuscitation and maintenance of organ perfusion, but late deaths from nosocomial infection and sequential multi-organ failure (MOF) remain high. Although bacterial infection is the commonest cause of septic shock[1], MOF may also result from endotoxaemia that follows haemorrhagic shock[2]. This is due to increased intestinal permeability which has been demonstrated in patients with burns, in patients following cardiopulmonary bypass and in patients with trauma. Bacterial translocation may be sporadic or frequent and the prevalence depends upon methods of detection and whether there is obstruction to the gastrointestinal tract. The still unproven proposition is that primary events such as shock, stress and vasoconstrictor drugs lead to mucosal barrier breakdown. Bowel rest, gastric pH neutralization[3], decreased intestinal peristalsis and non-selective antibiotic administration lead to bacterial overgrowth[4]. The combination of bacterial overgrowth, mucosal breakdown and increased intestinal permeability leads to translocation[5]. However, many serious and life-threatening infections may occur in the absence of such factors and the pathogenesis in such cases remains speculative.

Pathophysiology is discussed further in Chapter 1 and management of septic shock in Chapter 6. Essentially fluid resuscitation and maximizing oxygen delivery are the mainstay of treatment[6, 7]. Below are some of the main categories of pathogens causing systemic infection but there is some overlap between categories (e.g. viral infections and returning travellers with viral haemorrhagic fever) and with other chapters.

BACTERAEMIA

Bacteraemia is bacterial infection of the bloodstream which may be primary, where there is no obvious source, or secondary, arising as a complication of infection elsewhere such as pneumonia. The organisms responsible for bacteraemia may be Gram positive, Gram negative or fungi (may be referred to as fungaemia). Components of the cell wall of Gram-positive organisms such as teichoic acid act in the same way as the endotoxin of Gram-negative organisms to initiate release of the cytokine cascade with all the features of severe sepsis as discussed in Chapter 1.

Overall, infection occurs in 15–40% of all ICU admissions and the crude mortality rate lies between 10–80%, but this includes mortality from the underlying condition (see also the EPIC Study results referred to in Chapter 1, p.3). The incidence of bacteraemia and fungaemia in an adult intensive care unit (ICU) in the UK increased from 17.7 per 1000 admissions in 1985 to 80.3 per 1000 in 1996; 18% of episodes were community acquired and 82% hospital acquired[8]. Gram-positive and Gram-negative bacteria accounted for 46.9% and 31.5% of episodes, respectively. Polymicrobial infection accounted for 17.8% and fungal infection for 3.8% of episodes. *Staphylococcus aureus* (22.5%), *Staphylococcus epidermidis* (7.6%) and *Streptococcus pneumoniae* (7.9%) were the main Gram-positive bacteria identified whereas *Escherichia coli* (6%), *Enterobacter cloacae* (7%), *Klebsiella aerogenes* (3.8%), *Pseudomonas aeruginosa* (5.1%) and *Acinetobacter* spp. (3.8%) were the predominant Gram-negative organisms.

There has been a sustained rise in the incidence of serious infection due to multiply resistant Gram-positive organisms over the last decade[9] because of the increasing number of immunocompromised patients receiving intensive care, the use of more invasive monitoring and the use of broad-spectrum antimicrobial therapy, which eradicates most of the Gram-negative bacteria[10]. Control of infection is therefore a major challenge at present (see Chapter 3)[11].

INTRAVASCULAR CATHETER INFECTION

Aetiology

Coagulase-negative staphylococci, methicillin-resistant *S. aureus* (MRSA) and enterococci are the commonest nosocomial bloodstream pathogens[12]. Many nosocomial bloodstream infections are related to the use of intravascular devices. Invasive indwelling catheters such as arterial and central venous pressure (CVP) lines rapidly become colonized with micro-organisms often related to thrombosis in the cannula, and the incidence of colonization rises over time. The introduction of triple-lumen catheters with closed on–off taps may have reduced the incidence of colonization but the practice of rewiring catheters over a Seldinger wire remains controversial. Pulmonary artery catheters are subject to the same risks but in addition serious consequences such as right heart infective endocarditis may occur following endocardial damage. The rate of bacteraemia associated with CVP catheters is variably reported as 4–14% and with long-term cuffed silicone catheters ranges from 4–43%[13].

Diagnosis

A semi-quantitative technique is required by which, for example, the catheter is rolled across a blood agar plate and following incubation the colonies are counted (the Maki technique)[14]. There is increasing interest in the use of methods of diagnosis that do not require removal of the line such as sampling the tip whilst the catheter is *in situ* by means of a brush[15].

Management

Prevention of line-associated sepsis hinges upon aseptic insertion[16] and experienced personnel such as intravenous therapy teams in the hospital generally; both of which have been shown to be cost-effective. The practice of changing lines over a guidewire has recently been reviewed; exchange of CVP lines every 3 days over a wire was associated with a similar rate of infection as changing the lines when clinically indicated and the routine replacement of intravascular lines may increase the risk of bloodstream infection[17–19]. Routine culture from all catheters from patients in the ICU should be performed and, if this reveals colonization with the same organism as that from the bloodstream, the CVP should be removed and a new one inserted on the opposite side. The use of filters has not been shown to provide protection against catheter-related infection. However, there is evidence that the incidence of systemic infection associated with pulmonary artery catheters can be greatly reduced by removing the catheter within 4 days[20, 21]. Certainly the incidence of infection increases markedly beyond 72 hours and, even though the catheter must sometimes remain in place longer, ICU staff should be aware of the increased risk of infection.

Peripheral intravascular cannulae should be changed regularly every 48–72 hours, except where there are no alternative sites, and should be covered with a clear dressing through which thrombophlebitis can be diagnosed early. The use of topical antimicrobial preparations does lower the rate of catheter-related infection but there is a higher risk of *Candida* colonization and infection. Mupirocin reduces the risk of staphylococcal colonization of internal jugular lines but routine use may encourage the emergence of resistant *S. aureus*. Methods of prevention of infection associated with intravascular devices have recently been reviewed[22]. For short- but not long-term catherization, silver-impregnated subcutaneous collagen cuffs provide a potential antimicrobial deterrent. Other methods for incorporating silver into catheters await full development and evaluation. Coating catheters with antimicrobial agents inside and out (minocycline, rifampicin) reduces both colonization and catheter-related septicaemia[23].

The use of CVP catheters impregnated with either minocycline and rifampicin or chlorhexidine and silver sulfadiazine was recently compared with the use of unimpregnated catheters in the USA, where current estimates of bloodstream infection range from 4 to 13 per 1000 patient days[24] and attributable mortality from bloodstream infections is estimated at a rate of 25%[25]. Catheters impregnated with minocycline and rifampicin were one-third as likely to be colonized as catheters impregnated with chlorhexidine and silver sulfadiazine, and catheter-related infection was significantly less likely with catheters impregnated with minocycline and rifampicin than with those impregnated with chlorhexidine and silver sulfadiazine[26]. The reduction in infection is greatest in those who require vascular access for more than 7 days. This study has been criticized[27] but these and other studies emphasize that the use of antimicrobial-impregnated catheters should complement rather than replace adequate aseptic practice[26, 28–31]. These catheters cost about £35; their cost-effectiveness is estimated at an additional £750 to prevent one infection and £3000 to prevent one death[30].

Development and implementation of protocols for catheter care and changing policies may be effective locally in reducing the incidence of infections. Where the organism remains sensitive, Gram-positive infection can be treated with teicoplanin or vancomycin but there is an increasing risk of emergence of resistant strains. Rifampicin also has potent antistaphylococcal activity but resistance develops readily if it is used alone. Duration of treatment is controversial; 2 weeks is probably sufficient if the catheters can be removed, but where there is significant risk of endocarditis (e.g. with *S. aureus*) a longer period of treatment is wise. Drainage of suppurative collections should also be undertaken.

STAPHYLOCOCCAL INFECTION

Aetiology
Both *S. aureus* and coagulase-negative staphylococci such as *S. epidermidis* are skin commensals but *S. aureus* is more virulent. Thirty to fifty per cent of healthy adults are colonized with *S. aureus* and those colonized are at increased risk of invasive infection[32, 33]. Rates of colonization are high amongst type 1 diabetics, intravenous drug abusers, surgical patients and patients with AIDS. The increase in staphylococcal infections in recent years parallels the use of intravascular devices. Whether colonization leads to systemic infection depends on the virulence of the organism and host defence mechanisms. The commonest skin manifestation is impetigo but other lesions may arise by haematogenous spread of organisms or toxins during septicaemia. *S. epidermidis* is part of the normal skin flora but can cause serious infection in immunocompromised patients and those with intravascular cannulae and prosthetic devices such as pacemakers, heart valves and cerebrospinal fluid (CSF) shunts.

Invasive systemic infection
Invasive *S. aureus* infection may result in abscesses of the lung, kidney and bone. Lung abscesses are commonest in elderly debilitated patients, and in alcoholics and intravenous drug abusers who are prone to aspiration. The latter group is also at a high risk of endocarditis. Lung abscesses complicating staphylococcal pneumonia appear on the chest X-ray as multiple thin-walled cystic spaces containing little fluid, but classical *S. aureus* pneumonia with these features is now relatively unusual because of earlier and improved therapy. In patients with ventilator-associated pneumonia, chest X-ray appearances may be indistinguishable from those of Gram-negative pneumonia. Antibiotic treatment and physiotherapy should be continued for 2–4 weeks but surgical resection of severely damaged lung is occasionally necessary, although less so in recent years.

The mortality rate from staphylococcal bacteraemia is 11–43%; age greater than 50 years, a non-removable source of infection and serious cardiac, respiratory or neurological comorbidity are associated with a poor outcome. The mortality rate from nosocomial endocarditis may be as high as 56% and is highest in staphylococcal infection[32]. Bacteraemia due to MRSA has a higher mortality rate even after correction for severity of illness: 58% versus 32% in methicillin-sensitive bacteraemia[34,35].

Toxic shock syndrome

Staphylococcal and streptococcal toxic shock syndromes are characterized by rapid onset of high fever, shock, capillary leak and MOF. In both cases bacterial products induce excessive release of cytokines. The toxins released act as superantigens capable of simultaneously activating large numbers of T cells[36].

Presentation

Staphylococcal toxic shock syndrome was originally described in young women associated with the use of tampons but it is now recognized that it may also follow superficial skin lesions or wound infections. Strains, especially those belonging to phage group 1, gain access through the skin or vagina and produce toxins (toxic shock syndrome toxin-1 and enterotoxins) which cause diarrhoea, vomiting, fever, myalgia and rash with erythema of the skin and mucosae leading to desquamation (Plate 7). Streptococcal toxic shock syndrome due to *Streptococcus pyogenes* is now the more common condition and is also associated with muscle damage and tissue necrosis. A working group has defined a definite case as an illness with isolation of organisms from a normal sterile site with clinical signs[37].

Management

In addition to antibiotic treatment, hypovolaemia requires aggressive fluid resuscitation, and both shock and MOF require inotropic therapy and aggressive organ support (Chapter 6).

Ideally an antimicrobial agent that suppresses toxin production and kills the bacteria is preferred, hence earlier suggestions of clindamycin as the drug of choice[38]. However, the likelihood of clindamycin resistance emerging and the risk of diarrhoea has promoted the use of drug combinations such as flucloxacillin

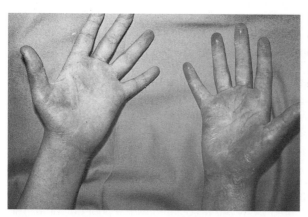

Plate 7 Desquamation of the palms of the hands, one of the later manifestations of toxic shock syndrome.

with gentamicin, which may also inhibit toxin production. Intravenous immuno-globulin may also be effective in neutralizing toxins in both staphylococcal and streptococcal syndromes[39].

Toxic epidermal necrolysis

This is a drug reaction with a high mortality rate which may mimic systemic sepsis or staphylococcal scalded skin syndrome. Sulphonamides, gold, phenytoin and allopurinol are implicated but the condition can also be precipitated by lymphoma and graft-versus-host disease. There may be a prodomal illness with malaise and fever followed by widespread tender blistering of the skin (Plate 8). Large areas of skin are easily rubbed off by minimal pressure. Fluid loss is high and septicaemia and pneumonia may occur secondarily requiring admission to the ICU. The diagnosis is clinical but the differential diagnosis includes staphylo-coccal scalded skin syndrome, which can be differentiated histologically by involvement of the whole epidermis in epidermal necrolysis. Management consists of fluid replacement and treatment of secondary infection.

PYREXIA OF UNKNOWN ORIGIN (PUO)

Not all patients with pyrexia have an infection and infection can, of course, occur in the absence of fever, particularly in the elderly in whom thermoregulatory responses are impaired due to disordered autonomic function, e.g. reduced ability to shiver to maintain temperature. PUO implies a temperature that does not resolve spontaneously and whose cause cannot be ascertained despite considerable diagnostic effort. The original definition which defined a minimum pyrexial period of 2 weeks is less applicable to patients requiring intensive care. Generally patients with PUO do not require admission to the ICU but the approach adopted below is often appropriate in patients with a persistent pyrexia present either on admission or afterwards.

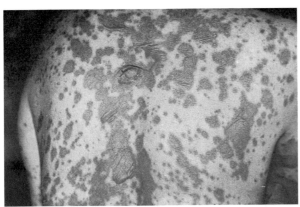

Plate 8 Toxic epidermal necrolysis. (Courtesy of Emond RTD et al. (1995). *Colour Atlas of Infectious Diseases*, 3rd edit. Mosby-Wolfe: London.)

Aetiology

In younger patients with PUO, fever is usually due to an infection, but in an older age group, neoplastic disease is as common a cause as infection. Connective tissue diseases and drug reactions occur at any age. The more chronic infections, which are difficult to diagnose, include infective endocarditis, biliary tract infection and infections with intracellular organisms such as *Salmonella* and *Brucella*. Tuberculosis (see Chapter 7), one of the commoner causes of PUO, should always be considered, as should a deep-seated abscess. Viral causes are less common and fungal infection is largely confined to immuno-suppressed patients (see Chapter 12). The commonest tumours causing PUO are lymphomas, but leukaemia and other solid tumours, particularly with hepatic metastases, may also be responsible.

Diagnosis

A thorough history (often from relatives if the patient is obtunded or heavily sedated) and careful examination are essential to guide investigation. A number of patterns of fever related to specific diagnoses have been described but this feature is relatively rare (e.g. malaria). Relative bradycardia occurs with some infections, including typhoid fever (see below), legionnaires' disease and brucellosis. The initial diagnostic evaluation should include the following:

1. Full blood count
2. Routine blood chemistry
3. Liver function tests
4. Urine analysis and culture
5. Autoimmune screen
6. Repeated blood and other cultures
7. Cytomegalovirus (CMV) IgM antibodies or virus detection in blood
8. Tuberculin skin test
9. Computed tomography (CT) or radionuclide scan of abdomen

Echocardiography or transoesophageal echo studies may be helpful if endocarditis is suspected. HIV testing and further investigation will depend on the background of the patient and any abnormalities identified by the above tests. Labelled leukocyte scanning may also be helpful to detect focal infection (see Chapter 4). Invasive procedures such as needle biopsy (liver or kidney), marrow aspiration, laparoscopy or, rarely, laparotomy may be necessary to confirm the diagnosis. Newer diagnostic tests have had little impact in making a successful diagnosis, hence the importance of a meticulous history and examination and as far as possible discontinuing existing drug treatment[40].

Factitious fever should be suspected when all other investigations repeatedly fail to identify a cause, but persistence is essential and repeated investigation for treatable neoplastic disease should be a priority. Management will be determined by the presumed (or confirmed) diagnosis and may include broad spectrum antimicrobial agents, antituberculous therapy or a trial of corticosteroids.

RETURNING TRAVELLERS

Particular problems may be presented by travellers returning from abroad. These patients may have an infective or non-infective cause for fever and, if infective, may have a fever characteristic of tropical disease. As well as a meticulous general history, details of dietary habits, sexual contacts, vaccination status, countries visited and adequacy of prophylaxis are all important. The time between the end of the period of travel and the onset of illness together with a knowledge of the incubation period for indigenous infections will give some idea of the possible differential diagnosis. For example, some viral diseases such as arboviruses and Marburg virus disease have short incubation periods of less than 2 weeks, whereas protozoal diseases such as visceral leishmaniasis have an incubation period of 6 weeks or more.

Repeated physical examination is necessary and a blood film should always be requested with the full blood count looking for malaria parasites and trypanosomiasis. The white blood cell (WBC) count usually shows leukocytosis in bacterial infections, but leukopenia is a feature of *Salmonella* and some viral infections, whereas eosinophilia is a feature of helminth infections. Blood cultures should be incubated for longer than normal to recover *Brucella*. Appropriate paired (baseline and 10 days later) serological tests should be done for syphilis, leptospirosis, rickettsial diseases, brucellosis, leishmaniasis, amoebiasis, trypanosomiasis, toxoplasmosis, filariasis and schistosomiasis if these seem likely from the clinical history and geographical area of travel. If a diagnosis remains elusive, marrow or liver biopsy should be performed. In some cases, however, treatment must be started empirically before the diagnosis is confirmed.

Salmonella infections

Salmonellae are non-lactose-fermenting Gram-negative bacteria responsible for the clinical syndromes of salmonellosis (gastroenteritis due to food poisoning) and enteric fever (typhoid and paratyphoid fever). Although there may be some overlap between these two clinical syndromes, such as the systemic spread of salmonellosis with bacteraemia, there are significant differences between the two (Table 8.1).

Enteric fever

The incubation period for infection caused by *Salmonella typhi* and *S. paratyphi* is about 10–14 days and the onset is usually characterized by fever, malaise, headache and respiratory symptoms including bronchitis. During the second week of symptoms, the fever may be as high as 40°C and indeed the patient may become quite toxic. Gastrointestinal symptoms may not be prominent and abdominal pain or constipation is more common than diarrhoea. The classical rash of rose spots is not always seen especially in dark-skinned individuals. The clinical symptoms of infection caused by *S. typhi* and *S. paratyphi* are similar. Enteric fever is relatively uncommon in the developed world but may be seen in

Table 8.1 Differences between enteric and non-enteric salmonellae.

Feature	Food poisoning	Enteric fever
Acquisition	Zoonosis (e.g. from poultry)	Human pathogen only
Disease	Gastroenteritis	Typhoid and paratyphoid fever
Outcome	Usually not life-threatening	Life-threatening
Geography	Worldwide including UK	In the UK and Europe, usually acquired from abroad
Antibiotics	Not usually required	Indicated
Example	*Salmonella enteritidis*	*Salmonella typhi*

the returned traveller, especially if she or he has recently been to Asia or Central or South America. Infection is usually acquired from ingestion of contaminated water, shellfish and unpasteurized milk. The majority of patients do not require admission to the ICU unless the clinical course is complicated by relapse (10–20% of cases), gastrointestinal perforation (0.5–5% of cases) or gastrointestinal haemorrhage (10–20% of cases)[41]. Disseminated infection including spread to the liver, bone and brain may also occur.

Diagnosis. Clinical suspicion of enteric fever in the pyrexial patient who has recently been abroad is important; the absence of gastrointestinal symptoms is not inconsistent with the diagnosis. The definitive diagnosis is made by isolation of the organism from blood cultures or bone marrow culture (most likely during the first week), faeces (second week) or other sites such as bile and urine. Although the Widal test may confirm a diagnosis retrospectively by detecting antibodies to somatic and flagellar antigens, previous exposure or vaccination against typhoid complicates interpretation and, because it may not be locally available, this test is less frequently used nowadays.

Management. Organ support such as renal replacement and ventilation are essential in the severely ill patient requiring admission to the ICU. The antimicrobial agent of choice is now ciprofloxacin (i.v., 400 mg 12-hourly) or chloramphenicol (i.v., 500 mg 6-hourly), but if the latter is chosen marrow toxicity should be monitored for by regular blood counts and blood antibiotic levels. The mortality rate from untreated cases may be as high as 30%, but in those given appropriate antimicrobial chemotherapy it is usually 5% or less. Predictors of a poor outcome include delirium and reduced consciousness at presentation, thrombocytopenia or complications such as perforation and peritonitis[42]. There is considerable concern at the international spread of multi-resistant strains and these now account for about 20% of all *S. typhi* isolates in the UK, mainly acquired from the Indian subcontinent; resistance does not seem to be a major problem in Africa, South or Central America[43]. Close liaison with public health authorities (this is a notifiable disease in the UK and in many other countries) and travel bureaux is essential to monitor the incidence and spread.

Salmonellosis

Food poisoning resulting in gastroenteritis is commonly caused by non-enteric serotypes of *Salmonella*. The most common serotypes encountered in the UK include *S. enteritidis*, *S. typhimurium*, *S. virchow* and *S. hadar*[44]. These bacteria are acquired from animals via the food chain, and such foodstuffs as meat, eggs and unpasteurized milk may be implicated. Certain serotypes are associated with particular animal sources such as *S. dublin* from cattle and *S. cholerae-suis* from pigs. Following the resolution of symptoms, major life-threatening complications or prolonged excretion of *Salmonella* are uncommon.

Presentation. The vast majority of patients with salmonellosis will not require ICU care. However, severely dehydrated patients who are in shock following severe diarrhoea, or patients who develop systemic *Salmonella* infection, may be admitted for organ support. It has recently been suggested that extraintestinal non-typhoid *Salmonella* be classified into four groups: primary and secondary bacteraemia, and digestive and non-digestive focal infection[45]. This facilitates the identification of risk factors (e.g. immunosuppression associated with primary bacteraemia), helps predict mortality and guide management strategies. Approximately 2% of patients with *Salmonella* gastroenteritis develop bacteraemia as a result of bacteria gaining access to the bloodstream via a damaged gastrointestinal tract. Some strains are more prone to cause bacteraemia than others and these include *S. dublin* (25%) and *S. cholerae-suis* (74%); in contrast, the incidence of bacteraemia acquired from *S. enteritidis* and *S. typhimurium* is only approximately 1%[45]. Disorders of cell-mediated immunity and treatment with corticosteroids are particular risk factors for bacteraemia[45, 46].

Diagnosis. Patients with systemic salmonellosis are clinically indistinguishable from those with severe sepsis, bacteraemia or septic shock, but a recent history of gastrointestinal symptoms may suggest the diagnosis. However, such a history may not be available because the patient is moribund or confused, such as may occur in the elderly. Stool, for routine culture, and blood cultures are essential for a microbiological diagnosis.

Management. Organ support including physiological fluid replacement and antibiotics is the key to effective management of the severely ill patient with systemic salmonellosis; uncomplicated salmonellosis is usually self-limiting and does not require antibiotics. Patients with severe diarrhoea, especially if bloody, and patients with *Salmonella* isolated from blood cultures or elsewhere (e.g. CSF) require intravenous antibiotics. Ciprofloxacin (i.v., 400 mg 12-hourly) is now the treatment of choice for *Salmonella* bacteraemia, chloramphenicol (i.v., 500 mg 6-hourly; toxic effects on the bone marrow should be monitored by regular blood counts and regular serum assays) or ceftriaxone (2–4 g once daily) are alternatives, depending on the results of susceptibility testing. The optimal duration of therapy is not known but a median duration of 17 days has been reported[47]. Intravenous antibiotics should probably be continued for a minimum of 7 days, especially in vulnerable or immunosuppressed patients, followed by oral therapy. As with *S. typhi* and *S. paratyphi*, there is increasing concern about antibiotic resistance which requires continuous worldwide surveillance to guide empirical therapy.

Malaria
Aetiology
Malaria is an acute febrile illness caused by *Plasmodium* parasites within red blood cells giving rise to the characteristic paroxysms of fever. *P. falciparum* is the most serious form and is associated with a significant mortality. Malaria is endemic in the tropics – the Americas, Asia, Africa and the Pacific area. In the UK and most of Europe malaria usually occurs only in tourists, people employed overseas, business travellers and immigrants. About 10 people each year die in Britain from malaria, usually due to *P. falciparum*. The increase in incidence of 'imported' malaria is due to a combination of factors: increased travel, increased resistance of *P. falciparum* to antimalarial drugs, delayed diagnosis and treatment, and neglected travel advice or poor compliance with prophylactic regimens.

The life cycle requires mosquitoes for transmission to humans; after the bite, parasites progress through the liver and red blood cells. Parasitized red blood cells are less flexible than normal and become sequestered in post-capillary venules of the brain, liver, spleen, kidneys and lung where disruption occurs with spread of merozoites, red cell products, malaria antigen and pigment into the local circulation, inducing further endothelial damage. Cerebral malaria results in coma and cerebral oedema, and acute renal tubular necrosis is common. However, blackwater fever due to acute massive intravascular haemolysis is now rare. Centrilobular necrosis occurs in the liver often with jaundice, partly due to haemolysis.

Presentation
An accurate history is crucially important; a brief visit to an endemic area may be sufficient for exposure to infection. Even in patients with acquired immunity, such as those reared in endemic areas, immunity is incomplete and wanes with time. Malaria should also be considered in the differential diagnosis of fever after blood transfusion, organ transplantation and needle stick injury[48]. The incubation period varies with the species. Headache, shivering, fever, myalgia, vomiting and weakness occur. Associated diarrhoea may cause dehydration and convulsions occur especially in children.

Diagnosis

The diagnosis is suspected on the basis of the characteristic clinical history in a patient who has lived in an endemic area or has travelled there recently, and is confirmed by repeated examination of thick and thin stained blood films for schizonts. A collateral history (i.e. from relative or partner) should be obtained in the comatose ICU patient. An antimalarial drug taken before a blood sample may temporarily clear the blood of parasites and so further blood films should be taken. Negative blood films reduce the likelihood of malaria and in particular the chance of progressing to complicated disease but do not exclude the diagnosis, and often treatment should be started if malaria remains the most likely diagnosis after excluding other causes. Expert help in species identification can be obtained from one of the tropical disease centres.

Haemoglobin concentration may fall and the reticulocyte count may also be low, indicating a degree of marrow suppression. The platelet count is often reduced but clotting is usually normal.

The differential diagnosis includes most of the other causes of acute sepsis but, when associated with renal failure, leptospirosis and viral haemorrhagic fevers should be considered. When the patient presents with coma, meningitis and encephalitis should be excluded. Jaundice accompanying fever makes yellow fever, typhus, biliary sepsis and leptospirosis more likely but septicaemia can manifest with any of these as an indicator of organ dysfunction.

Management

Management consists of eliminating the parasites with drugs, supportive measures, and recognition and management of complications[48]. The British National Formulary (BNF) or local equivalent should be consulted for details of appropriate drug combinations for treatment of the various forms of malaria and for prophylaxis for travellers. Chloroquine is indicated for P. vivax, P. ovale, P. malariae and P. falciparum malaria, and for P. vivax and P. ovale, primaquine should be added. P. falciparum malaria may be resistant to chloroquine and therefore the more toxic quinine should be given parenterally. Quinine alone will not cure P. falciparum malaria, but an alternative drug combination such as Fansidar (pyrimethamine with sulphonamide) may suffice, although resistance is becoming more common. Primaquine should not be given to patients who are at risk of glucose-6-phosphate dehydrogenase deficiency, otherwise severe haemolysis may be precipitated and this should therefore be screened for first. The presence of renal or hepatic dysfunction requires modification of the drug dose and/or dosing interval.

Patients with P. falciparum malaria are unlikely to respond to chloroquine and unless they have the severe form should be treated with:

1. quinine sulphate, 600 mg 8-hourly, with a single oral dose of pyrimethamine–sulfadoxine (Fansidar) of three tablets. The latter is contraindicated if there is a history of sulphonamide sensitivity. If resistance to Fansidar is suspected then doxycycline, 200 mg once and then 100 mg daily for 6 days, should be given except for children under 8 years of age and pregnant women;
   or

2. mefloquine, 20 mg base kg^{-1} to a maximum of 1500 mg divided into two doses 6 hours apart. This is contraindicated in pregnancy, in people taking β-blocking drugs and where there is a history of psychiatric disease including epilepsy;

   or

3. halofantrine, 500 mg 6-hourly for three doses and repeated after 1 week.

Whilst patients are being treated it is important to monitor the efficacy of the treatment, observe for developing complications and anticipate drug toxicity. *P. falciparum* malaria should be regarded as severe if parasitaemia is greater than 2% or if complications such as cerebral malaria, renal failure, acute respiratory distress syndrome (ARDS), disseminated intravascular coagulation (DIC), hyperpyrexia or jaundice occur.

Patients with malaria in the ICU are likely to require control of convulsions, correction of hypoglycaemia (which is more common in children and pregnant women) and organ support, particularly renal replacement therapy. Whole blood exchange or plasmapheresis is useful if more than 10% of red blood cells are parasitized and when complications worsen. Rehydration therapy is often required and, in view of the risk of multiple organ failure, requires monitoring with a central venous pressure or pulmonary artery catheter. Convulsions are common and require correction of contributing factors such as hypoglycaemia, as well as anti-convulsants. Treatment of cerebral malaria with dexamethasone should also be considered. Consultation with an infectious disease physician or an expert in tropical medicine is generally advisable, especially in complicated cases.

Patients with cerebral malaria require intravenous therapy with quinine to achieve maximum blood levels as quickly but safely as possible. Quinidine is an acceptable alternative until quinine becomes available. One of the following regimens is suitable:

1. quinine hydrochloride, 7 mg kg^{-1} loading dose to a maximum of 490 mg given over 30 minutes by i.v. infusion, which should be omitted if the patient has received quinine, quinidine or mefloquine in the preceding 24 hours. This is followed immediately by 10 mg kg^{-1} (maximum 700 mg) diluted in 10 ml kg^{-1} isotonic fluid by i.v. infusion over 4 hours, repeated at intervals of 8 hours until the patient can take oral quinine, when 10 mg kg^{-1} to a maximum of 700 mg is given 8-hourly to complete a 7-day course of treatment;

   or

2. quinine dihydrochloride, 20 mg kg^{-1} loading dose to a maximum of 1400 mg infused i.v. over 4 hours, omitted if the patient has received quinine, quinidine or mefloquine in the preceding 24 hours, and then continued as above;

   or

3. quinidine gluconate, 10 mg kg^{-1} (maximum 700 mg) loading dose i.v. infusion over 2 hours followed by 0.02 mg kg^{-1} min^{-1} (maximum 1.4 mg min^{-1}) for 72 hours or until the patient can swallow, then continue quinine as above;

   or

4. quinidine gluconate, 15 mg kg^{-1} loading dose i.v. over 4 hours, then after an interval of 4 hours infuse 7.5 mg kg^{-1} (maximum 525 mg) over 4 hours and repeat 8-hourly until oral quinine can be given.

A series of errors contributing to death from malaria has been identified which includes failure to take prophylaxis because of public ignorance, inconsistent advice or drug resistance, failure to diagnose or late diagnosis, unusual presentation or route of infection, and inadequate or insufficient blood films. These factors will lead to a delay in admission to hospital and start of treatment. It is essential to use the right drug, the right dose and route of administration and to monitor closely for complications, treating them as soon as they arise. CT scanning is preferred to lumbar puncture to exclude other causes of encephalopathy and certainly in the presence of raised intracranial pressure. If there is doubt about bacterial meningitis, empirical antibiotic treatment should be started.

Viral haemorrhagic fevers
These are severe and life-threatening diseases caused by a range of viruses which include Lassa fever, Ebola virus and Marburg virus. Outbreaks occur in West Africa (e.g. Nigeria, Sierra Leone) and patients may return to Europe either during the incubation period or with an illness at the port of entry suggestive of one these infections. These are multi-system infections which may present with fever, headache, malaise, diarrhoea, skin rashes (e.g. morbilliform), jaundice and organ failure. These viruses are considered to be very infectious and transmission to health care workers has been described.

Ideally, patients suspected of having one of these illnesses should be transferred to a high-security infectious disease unit but this is not always possible or feasible due to a delayed diagnosis or even a misdiagnosis. However, an infectious disease physician should be consulted on suspicion of a diagnosis and the laboratory informed as specimens should be processed as high risk. Although viral haemorrhagic fever is happily quite rare, it should be considered in the differential diagnosis of the returned traveller from Africa with a fever of undetermined origin.

OBSTETRIC INFECTIONS

Aetiology
Infection remains an important cause of maternal mortality[49]. In addition to those infections that occur in the general population, there are specific immunological and other features of pregnancy that alter the mother's response to infection[50], although most serious infections occur postpartum. Pregnancy is occasionally associated with disseminated viral infections such as herpes and there may also be increased susceptibility to the harmful effect of endotoxin. Asymptomatic bacteriuria is common and should be treated, as the risk of

pyelonephritis is high. The vagina and lower cervix normally contain aerobic and anaerobic bacteria and these together with other pathogens can spread during labour into the upper genital tract following premature rupture of membranes, instrumentation, or termination of pregnancy. If ascending infection occurs in the antenatal period, chorio-amnionitis may result. Following birth the commonest site of infection is the placental site leading to endometritis, but spread to the peritoneum can also occur. Wound infection of the episiotomy site or Caesarean section scar are less serious events. Infection is often poly-microbial and includes anaerobes (*Bacteroides, Clostridium*), Enterobacteriaceae (*E. coli, Klebsiella, Enterobacter*), β-haemolytic streptococci (group A and B), *Chlamydia* and *Mycoplasma*. Organisms such as *Listeria monocytogenes* and group A streptococci can cause infection by haematogenous spread, and mastitis due to staphylococci or streptococci can be severe in lactating women. Opportunistic infections should raise the possibility of HIV infection.

Septic shock caused by streptococci can produce a devastating illness with death occurring within hours (see above). β-Haemolytic group A streptococci (*S. pyogenes*) may cause toxic shock syndrome (pyrogenic exotoxin A) and, with anaerobes, necrotizing fasciitis. The mortality rate from necrotizing fasciitis may be higher where it arises in the pelvis compared with other body sites. Intravenous benzylpenicillin (2.4 g 4–6-hourly) and clindamycin (600 mg 6-hourly) should be started immediately; despite the risk of inducing *Clostridium difficile* infection clindamycin has good antianaerobic activity and penetrates soft tissues in high concentrations. Toxic shock syndrome due to *S. aureus* is less common in pregnancy and usually follows septic abortion or other instrumentation.

Diagnosis

In addition to the usual septic screen (e.g. blood, urine, sputum, etc., cultures), specimens of tissue from uterine aspiration (or taken during surgery) should be sent to the laboratory for aerobic and anaerobic culture. Persistent sepsis or deterioration after delivery may be due to a localized abscess, resistant organisms or the development of pelvic thrombophlebitis. Pelvic X-rays may show gas in the tissue planes, i.e. gas gangrene, which is usually a fulminating illness with renal failure, profound coagulopathy and extreme hypotension. Septic pelvic thrombophlebitis may be diagnosed by CT or magnetic resonance imaging (MRI), and requires aggressive antibiotic therapy and anticoagulation. Persistent sepsis despite these measures may require surgery for venous ligation or excision.

Management

The management of septic shock in pregnancy is similar to that in the non-pregnant patient but the fetus may be adversely affected by a profound metabolic acidosis or the side-effects of antibiotics, especially during the first trimester[51]. The effects of inotropes on the placental circulation in undelivered mothers also require careful evaluation. Broad-spectrum intravenous antibiotic cover (e.g. cefotaxime, 1–2 g 8-hourly, and metronidazole, 500 mg 8-hourly) should be started immediately but surgery and the early delivery of the fetus is often required. Management of gas gangrene involves high-dose intravenous benzylpenicillin (2.4 g 4–6-hourly) and urgent laparotomy for hysterectomy and excision of all gangrenous tissue. The same approach with aggressive surgical debridement is required for necrotizing fasciitis.

VIRAL INFECTIONS

Serious viral infections requiring admission to the ICU usually occur in immuno-compromised patients (see Chapter 12) and those with underlying chronic cardiopulmonary disease[52]. These may be subdivided in those of the respiratory tract (see Chapter 7), skin and associated tissues, and generalized infection.

Influenza A and B
Aetiology
Influenza affects all age groups but is more severe in the elderly and those with chronic underlying diseases such as diabetes, chronic obstructive airway disease and immunosuppression. Bacterial superinfection may occur, giving rise to a biphasic illness with a concomitant increase in mortality.

Diagnosis
This is made by viral culture of respiratory secretions, throat swab, tracheal sputum or bronchoscopic specimens. Viral culture on transport media are required and a dry swab will not suffice. Rapid immunofluorescence techniques have a sensitivity of about 85% and a specificity greater than 90%. Serological tests are not immediately helpful as many patients do not develop IgM antibody, but they should be carried out to assist in making a diagnosis and for epidemiological purposes.

Management
Amantadine (100 mg twice daily for 7 days; reduced to 100 mg daily for patients over 65 years) should be used if the diagnosis of influenza A is made early, i.e. within 2 days of the onset of symptoms. Ribavirin may be given for influenza B. Killed influenza vaccine is 60–80% effective in preventing the disease and reducing mortality rates and should be administered to all at-risk groups and all patients over 75 years of age. Newer agents are now becoming available, but these need to be fully evaluated before widespread use[53], even in the critically ill patient.

Other respiratory viruses
Respiratory syncytial virus and adenovirus may cause severe pneumonia in immunocompetent patients and should be actively considered in the immuno-compromised patient with lower respiratory tract infection. Clinical features include fever, cough, pharyngitis and rhinitis with patchy diffuse infiltrates on the chest X-ray.

Diagnosis

Culture takes 2–3 weeks and serology may be negative as there are many different serotypes, but the antigen detection techniques now available are useful.

Management

There is no definitive treatment available for adenovirus except supportive care but isolated case reports suggest some benefit from high-dose intravenous immunoglobulin therapy in immunocompromised patients. Aerosolized ribavirin is used for the treatment of respiratory syncytial virus infection with variable success.

Varicella-zoster virus

About 15% of adult patients with this infection will develop pneumonia which has a high mortality rate (10–30%), especially during pregnancy.

Presentation

Patients present with a vesicular rash with respiratory symptoms developing 1–6 days later. Clinical examination of the chest and X-ray are often unremarkable although the radiological infiltrates can be nodular. Apart from pneumonia, other serious complications include secondary bacterial infection, cerebellar ataxia and encephalitis[54].

Diagnosis

This is largely clinical but can be confirmed by viral culture of vesicle fluid.

Management

Aciclovir (10 mg kg^{-1} 8-hourly) for at least 7 days is recommended. Consideration should be given to the possibility of occupational acquisition by non-immune staff (see Chapter 3) and the risk of acquisition by other non-immune patients, especially if immunocompromised.

Herpes simplex
Aetiology

This virus has a predilection for squamous epithelial sites in normal and immunocompromised hosts. Burns, radiation, smoking and traumatic intubation may predispose to infection of the lower respiratory tract and both the airways and lung parenchyma may be involved. Pneumonia may arise by aspiration or haematogenous spread in the immunocompromised host but is rare in the normal patient.

Diagnosis

There are no specific features to distinguish herpes simplex from other viral pneumonias except the characteristic vesicular features on bronchoscopy. Bronchoscopic specimens should be sent for culture (see Chapter 7) but the diagnosis can be confirmed only by finding cytological evidence of herpes simplex virus in lower respiratory tract specimens, as a positive culture may just indicate spread from mucocutaneous lesions in the absence of pneumonia.

Management
Aciclovir, 5–10 mg kg^{-1} 8-hourly, should be administered for 7–10 days.

Viral hepatitis
Aetiology
The major viral pathogens include hepatitis A, B, C, D, E and lately G. Patients requiring ICU admission will be those with liver failure. Epstein–Barr virus, other viral (e.g. CMV) and non-viral (e.g. leptospirosis) causes should always be considered in the differential diagnosis. Few patients with hepatitis A develop liver failure. Hepatitis B transmission occurs parenterally in intravenous drug users, by sexual contact and placental transfer. Hepatitis B virus is responsible for up to 75% of viral causes of fulminant hepatic failure and is a leading cause of chronic hepatitis, cirrhosis and hepatocellular carcinoma[55]. Hepatitis B is more common in adults and may be severe in pregnant women. Hepatitis C virus is an RNA virus which causes 90% of transfusion-related and 60% of sporadic cases of non-A, non-B hepatitis. Chronic liver disease occurs in 50% of patients with hepatitis C and 20% of them develop cirrhosis. Antibody to hepatitis C is found in 1–2% of patients in developed countries but in as many as 15% of the population in Egypt, partly due to the previous use of contaminated needles[56]. Alcohol consumption and older age at infection may result in an accelerated course. Hepatitis D occurs simultaneously with acute hepatitis B or causes superinfection in a chronic carrier of hepatitis B surface antigen. Hepatitis D virus commonly causes chronic hepatitis and 75% of these patients develop cirrhosis. Hepatitis E virus is a small RNA virus which causes sporadic, epidemic non-A, non-B hepatitis. It is transmitted by the faecal–oral route with the possibility of occasional parenteral transmission. Hepatitis G is a recently recognized virus transmitted by blood transfusion or parenteral exposure; it is not clear whether it results in any liver disease. The availability recently of an immunoblot assay for diagnosis suggests that the seroprevalence may be as high as 15–27% in some groups[57].

Presentation
The majority of patients with clinical evidence of hepatitis develop ill-defined malaise, raised levels of transaminases and jaundice. When fulminant liver failure occurs, management in the ICU is essential.

Diagnosis
There is an increasing range of serological and molecular techniques available to confirm the aetiology and indicate the stage or severity of hepatitis. Some of these are routine, e.g. surface antigen for hepatitis B, antibody for hepatitis A, whilst others are more complex and available only in certain centres, e.g. polymerase chain reaction (PCR) for hepatitis C. These should be discussed with a virologist or microbiologist and arranged appropriately.

Management

Treatment of viral hepatitis is often supportive but prevention by vaccination is very important. All health care workers at risk for occupational exposure should be vaccinated against hepatitis B (see Chapter 3).

Cytomegalovirus
Aetiology

CMV rarely if ever causes infection in the normal host that requires ICU care. Donor allografts are the source of infection in virtually all cases of kidney, heart, lung and bone marrow transplants. Although the incidence of CMV infection in transplanted patients is high, many patients remain asymptomatic. Risk factors for symptomatic disease include primary infection, receipt of antithymocyte or antilymphocyte antibodies for the treatment of graft rejection, bone marrow transplant recipients with graft-versus-host disease, total body irradiation and age >50 years[58].

Presentation

The infection presents with fever, malaise and anorexia and often resembles infectious mononucleosis. The disease is normally mild but in the immuno-compromised host who develops primary infection, reinfection or secondary infection the course is more serious. Leukopenia and thrombocytopenia are common, hepatitis may occur, and in the case of liver transplant patients a biopsy is therefore required. Other gastrointestinal features include ulceration, abdominal pain and haemorrhage. Interstitial pneumonitis, likely to require intensive care, has a high mortality rate (80–90%)[52]. Retinitis, transverse myelitis, encephalitis (see Chapter 11) and cutaneous ulceration occur and superinfection with bacteria or fungi is a significant problem because of the additional immunosuppressive effects of CMV infection.

Diagnosis

Antigen detection combined with viral culture, i.e. detection of early antigen fluorescent foci (DEAFF), is the most rapid routine diagnostic method in widespread use but PCR is becoming available. Serology is primarily used for screening for initial susceptibility because of the significant time lag between infection and serological response. False-positive serological results may be obtained in patients who have received immunoglobulin, blood or plasma and false-negative results may occur in the patient unable to mount an antibody reaction. The virus may be cultured from virtually any tissue but a positive culture does not necessarily imply infection, as CMV may be shed in asymptomatic patients or in patients with symptoms due to another cause.

Management

All transplant or other patients with CMV should have their immunosuppressive therapy reduced if possible, e.g. lowering the dose of corticosteroids unless this compromises other aspects of their care. Ganciclovir is 100 times more active against CMV than aciclovir and studies in solid-organ transplant patients have shown that this agent reduces the morbidity of CMV compared with historical controls. The dose is $5-6\,mg\,kg^{-1}\,day^{-1}$, often administered as two infusions for 14–21 days, but this should be reduced in patients with renal insufficiency. After bone marrow transplantation the response to ganciclovir is not as good and combinations with CMV antiserum or foscarnet should be considered.

HIV infection
Aetiology
AIDS was originally described in 1981 as an epidemic of *Pneumocystis carinii* pneumonia in homosexual men (see also Chapter 12) The CD4 cell count (subset of circulating lymphocytes) and viral count are now used to stage HIV infection. In the early stages of the disease, asymptomatic lymphadenopathy occurs, and then pneumonia, idiopathic thrombocytopenia, herpes zoster or pulmonary tuberculosis may occur. These are all recognized complications of HIV infection and sometimes occur when the CD4 count (normally $600-1400\,mm^{-3}$) is relatively high ($200-500$ cells mm^{-3}). As the CD4 count falls, complications become increasingly frequent but life-threatening episodes are rare until the cell count falls to $<50\,mm^{-3}$. Patients with HIV are most likely to require intensive care for pulmonary infection, CNS infection and systemic bacterial sepsis during the later stages of their illness.

Early in the disease *S. pneumoniae* and *Haemophilus influenzae* are common pathogens. *P. carinii* occurred in 80% of patients before the use of prophylaxis but is much less common now. Tuberculosis should be considered particularly in intravenous drug users. CNS infections such as *Toxoplasma* occur relatively late and are less likely to require intensive care. Lymphoma, cryptococcal meningitis and dementia must also be considered in the differential diagnosis of a neurological presentation.

Diagnosis
A protocol to establish the presence of the most likely pathogens should be followed and should include bronchoscopy or bronchoalveolar lavage. Tracheal expectorated sputum, induced sputum or bronchoscopic specimens provide the diagnosis in the majority of cases. Lumbar puncture and MRI will be required for diagnosis of CNS involvement. However, the survival and prognosis continues to improve; a recent UK observational study indicated that, compared with patients diagnosed before 1987, those diagnosed after this year lived longer, especially if their initial diagnosis was not associated with *P. carinii* infection[59].

Management
P. carinii pneumonia should be treated with trimethoprim–sulphamethoxazole (see Chapters 5 and 7) or pentamidine, and patients with severe hypoxaemia should receive corticosteroids. Tuberculosis is a significant problem because of multiply resistant strains in some centres which pose major challenges to infection control. Patients should be started on a combination of drugs such as isoniazid, rifampicin, ethambutol and pyrazinamide. However, full consultation with the infectious disease or genitourinary physician is required as the treatment

of the underlying HIV disease is increasingly complex[60] and the potential for drug interactions great.

FUNGAL INFECTION

Fungal infections have increased in patients in ICUs in recent years and contribute significantly to morbidity and mortality in seriously ill patients[61]. Patients who receive antibiotics have an increased risk of oral and enteric colonization with *Candida albicans*, and administration of antacids also facilitates increased growth of *Candida* in the stomach. Virulence factors include the ability to attach to endothelial and epithelial cells, blunting the host response and the ability to secrete enzymes, facilitating tissue invasion. It seems likely that the gastrointestinal tract is an important source of *Candida* entering the bloodstream by fungal translocation especially where mucosal ischaemia exists.

Disseminated candidiasis
Presentation
This condition occurs after haematogenous spread of *Candida* to multiple organs resulting in the formation of microabscesses. Focal necrosis then occurs leading eventually to fatal organ dysfunction. The brain, heart, kidneys and the eye are most commonly affected. Ocular involvement, which often goes undetected, is an indication for systemic therapy. Even in asymptomatic patients, the presence of *Candida* in more than one blood culture should not be ignored and ophthalmoscopy should therefore be carried out regularly in patients at risk. *Candida* intravascular line infection should always be excluded in patients with positive blood cultures by removing the catheter tip for culture.

In critically ill patients a number of risk factors have been identified for development of haematogenous candidiasis:

1. The isolation of *Candida* spp. from skin, urine or mucosa
2. Treatment with two or more antibacterial agents
3. Immunosuppression or cytotoxic therapy
4. Parenteral nutrition

Diagnosis
Two or more sets of blood cultures should be sent as discussed in Chapter 4. There is little value in sending more than six sets of blood cultures. Serological tests are of limited value owing to the high incidence of false-negative results, especially in immunosuppressed patients. In the future PCR may help improve laboratory confirmation (see Chapter 4). A good clinical guide is the presence of *Candida* endophthalmitis which may lead to blindness if not treated.

Management
Amphotericin B (i.v., 0.5–1.5 mg kg^{-1} day^{-1} for a period of 14 days) is the drug of choice, with fluconazole (i.v., 400 mg day^{-1} or higher) as an alternative. It

should also be borne in mind that not all species of *Candida* are always fluconazole sensitive, e.g. *C. krusei*[62], and confirmation of the species with or without susceptibility testing may be required. Amphotericin B is the 'gold standard' antifungal agent but unfortunately it is potentially nephrotoxic and leads to electrolyte disturbances. Recently new formulations with less nephrotoxicity have become available[63]. AmBisone contains the active drug in a bilayer of liposomes and this preparation has been shown to be effective against invasive fungal infections including *Aspergillus* without significant renal impairment. A recent study in neutropenic patients demonstrated fewer breakthrough fungal infections and a lower incidence of toxicity in patients on liposomal amphotericin B (AmBisome) compared with conventional amphotericin B[64]. Other preparations of amphotericin B as a lipid complex or a colloidal dispersion are non-liposomal lipid preparations which have not been as extensively assessed in clinical trials. New preparations are, however, much more expensive than conventional preparations and should be used in patients with invasive systemic fungal infection who have renal impairment or in patients with documented invasive infection not responding to conventional amphotericin B in appropriate doses. Central venous catheters should be removed to eliminate a nidus of infection, and where there is evidence of infection in several organs 5-fluocytosine, which has good pharmacokinetic properties, may be added to amphotericin B but serum levels of 5-fluocytosine should be measured. Endocarditis is particularly common in patients with prosthetic valves; intravenous drug abuse and central venous catheters are predisposing factors. Surgical valve replacement or repair is essential to prevent death from embolization or cardiac failure.

Non-haematogenous candidiasis

If *Candida* is present at more than one site this may be an indication for systemic therapy. Oral nystatin usually eradicates oral *Candida*, but oesophageal lesions should be treated with fluconazole or amphotericin B. *Candida* is frequently implicated in polymicrobial intra-abdominal infection. Patients with risk factors for systemic infection should receive systemic antifungal therapy (see above). Treatment of candiduria in patients with an indwelling urinary catheter is not routinely recommended, but replacing or removing the catheter should be considered. Bladder irrigation with amphotericin B ($50mg\,l^{-1}$ in sterile water by continuous irrigation or intermittent infusions for 5–7 days) will reduce the urine counts but may not eradicate *Candida* without catheter removal. Candiduria in a patient without a catheter or local skin infection (e.g. balanitis) may be a manifestation of systemic candidiasis.

Other fungal infections

Other fungal infections are less common in the ICU but outbreaks of *Aspergillus* spp. have been reported where building work is being undertaken[65]. Invasive *Aspergillus* is primarily a respiratory infection, especially in neutropenic patients, and organisms may spread elsewhere from this site. Invasive *Aspergillus* should be treated with amphotericin B. Itraconazole is an alternative but is less effective. Fluconazole is not active against *Aspergillus*. Surgical resection of localized pulmonary disease (aspergilloma) may be necessary on occasion.

Mucormycosis may also occasionally present in diabetics or patients with haematological malignancies and requires antifungal therapy and aggressive surgical debridement. Dimorphic fungi such as *Histoplasma*, relatively common in North America, are uncommon in Europe.

Key points

- Late deaths from nosocomial infection and sequential multi-organ failure in critically ill patients remain high.
- Overall infection occurs in 15–40% of all ICU admissions and the crude mortality rate lies between 10 and 80%.
- Coagulase-negative staphylococci, MRSA and enterococci are the commonest nosocomial bloodstream pathogens.
- The increase in incidence of 'imported' malaria is due to a combination of factors: increased travel, increased resistance of *P. falciparum* to antimalarial drugs, delayed diagnosis and treatment, and neglected travel advice or poor compliance with prophylactic regimens.
- Septic shock caused by streptococci can produce a devastating illness with death occurring within hours.
- Fungal infections have increased in patients in ICUs in recent years and contribute significantly to morbidity and mortality in seriously ill patients.
- Amphotericin B is the 'gold standard' antifungal agent but unfortunately it is potentially nephrotoxic and leads to electrolyte disturbances.

REFERENCES

1. Astiz ME, Rackow EC (1998) Septic shock. *Lancet* **351**: 1501.
2. Rush BF, Sori AJ, Murphy TF *et al.* (1988) Endotoxemia and bacteremia during hemorrhagic shock: the link between trauma and sepsis? *Annals of Surgery* **207**: 549–554.
3. Driks MR, Craven DE, Celli BR *et al.* (1987) Nosocomial pneumonia in intubated patients given sucralfate as compared with antacids or histamine type 2 blockers. *New England Journal of Medicine* **317**: 1376–1382.
4. Deitch EA (1990) The role of intestinal barrier failure and bacterial translocation in the development of systemic infection and multiple organ failure. *Archives of Surgery* **125**: 403–404.
5. Romand J-A (1996) Bacterial translocation in the critically ill. *Current Opinion in Critical Care* **2**: 371–374.
6. Hayes MA, Timmins AC, Yau EHS *et al.* (1995) Elevation of systemic oxygen delivery in the treatment of the critically ill. *New England Journal of Medicine* **330**: 1717–1722.

7. Boyd O, Grounds RM, Bennett ED (1993) The beneficial effect of supranormalization of oxygen delivery with dopexamine hydrochloride on perioperative mortality. *Journal of the American Medical Association* **270**: 2699–2707.

8. Crowe M, Ispani P, Humphreys H *et al.* (1998) Bacteraemia in the adult intensive care unit of a teaching hospital in Nottingham, UK, 1985–1996. *European Journal of Clinical Microbiology and Infectious Diseases* **17**: 377–384.

9. Schaberg DR, Culver DH, Gaines KP (1991) Major trends in the microbial etiology of nosocomial infection. *American Journal of Medicine* **91** (Suppl 3B): 72S–75S.

10. Martin MA (1993) Nosocomial infections in intensive care units: an overview of their epidemiology, outcome and prevention. *New Horizons* **1**: 162–171.

11. Goldmann DA, Weinstein RA, Wenzel RP *et al.* (1996) Strategies to prevent and control the emergence and spread of anti-microbial-resistant micro-organisms in hospitals. A challenge to hospital leadership. *Journal of the American Medical Association* **275**: 234–240.

12. Bjornson HS (1993) Pathogenesis, prevention and management of catheter-associated infections. *New Horizons* **1**: 271–278.

13. Adal KA, Farr BM (1996) Central venous catheter-related infections: a review. *Nutrition* **112**: 208–213.

14. Maki DG, Weise CE, Sarafin HW (1977) A semi-quantitative culture method for identifying intravenous-catheter-related infection. *New England Journal of Medicine* **296**: 1305–1309.

15. Raad I (1998) Intravascular catheter-related infections. *Lancet* **351**: 893–898.

16. Raad I, Hohn DC, Gilbeath BJ *et al.* (1994) Prevention of central venous catheter-related infections by using maximal sterile barrier precautions during insertion. *Infection Control and Hospital Epidemiology* **15**: 231–238.

17. Cyna AM, Hovenden JL, Lehmann A *et al.* (1998) Routine replacement of central venous catheters: telephone survey of intensive care units in mainland Britain. *British Medical Journal* **316**: 1944–1945.

18. Cook D, Randolph A, Kernerman P *et al.* (1997) Central venous pressure catheter replacement strategies: a systematic review of the literature. *Critical Care Medicine* **25**: 1417–1424.

19. Cobb DK, High KP, Sawyer RG *et al.* (1991) A controlled trial of scheduled replacement of central venous and pulmonary artery catheters. *New England Journal of Medicine* **327**: 1062–1068.

20. Raad I, Umphrey J, Khan A *et al.* (1993) The duration of placement as a predictor of peripheral and pulmonary artery catheter infections. *Journal of Hospital Infection* **23**: 17–26.

21. Cohen Y, Fosse JP, Karoubi P *et al.* (1998) The 'hands off' catheter and the prevention of systemic infections associated with pulmonary artery catheters. A prospective study. *American Journal of Respiratory and Critical Care Medicine* **157**: 234–257.

22. Raad I, Darouiche R (1996) Prevention of infections associated with intravascular devices. *Current Opinion in Critical Care* **2**: 361–365.

23. Maki DG, Stolz SM, Wheeler S *et al.* (1997) Prevention of central venous catheter-related blood stream infection by use of an antiseptic-impregnated catheter. A randomised, controlled trial. *Annals of Internal Medicine* **127**: 257–266.

24. National Nosocomial Infections Surveillance (NNIS) System Report (1998) Data summary from October 1986–April 1998, issued June 1998. *American Journal of Infection Control* **26**: 522–533.

25. Wenzel RP (1998) Attributable mortality – the promise of better antimicrobial therapy. *Journal of Infectious Diseases* **178**: 917–919.

26. Darouiche RO, Raad I, Heard SO *et al.* (1999) A comparison of two antimicrobial-impregnated central venous catheters. *New England Journal of Medicine* **340**: 1–8.

27. Bach A (1999) Antimicrobial-impregnated central venous catheters. *New England Journal of Medicine* **340**: 1761.

28. Pearson ML (1996) Hospital Infection Control Practices Advisory Committee. Guidelines for prevention of intravascular device-related infections I. *American Journal of Infection Control* **24**: 262–277.

29. Pearson ML (1996) Hospital Infection Control Practices Advisory Committee. Guidelines for prevention of intravascular device-related infections II. *American Journal of Infection Control* **24**: 277–293.

30. Wenzel RP, Edmond MB (1999) The evolving technology of venous access. *New England Journal of Medicine* **340**: 48–50.

31. Elliott TSJ (1999) Role of antimicrobial central venous catheters for the prevention of associated infections. *Journal of Antimicrobial Chemotherapy* **43**: 441–446.

32. Lowy FD (1998) *Staphylococcus aureus* infections. *New England Journal of Medicine* **339**: 520–532.

33. Wenzel RP, Perl TM (1995) The significance of nasal carriage of *Staphylococcus aureus* and the incidence of postoperative wound infection. *Journal of Hospital Infection* **31**: 13–24.

34. Romero-Vivas J, Rubio M, Fernandez C *et al.* (1995) Mortality associated with nosocomial bacteremia due to methicillin-resistant *Staphylococcus aureus*. *Clinical Infectious Diseases* **21**: 1417–1423.

35. Blot S, Vandewoude K, Colardyn F (1998) *Staphylococcus aureus* infections. *New England Journal of Medicine* **339**: 2025–2027.

36. Troillet N, Samore MH (1998) Staphylococcal and streptococcal toxic shock syndromes. *Current Opinion in Critical Care* **4**: 282–287.

37. Working Group on Severe Streptococcal Infections (1993) Defining the group A streptococcal toxic shock syndrome: rationale and consensus definition. *Journal of the American Medical Association* **269**: 390–391.

38. Stevens DL (1996) The toxic shock syndromes. *Infectious Disease Clinics of North America* **10**: 727–746.

39. Stevens DL (1998) Rationale for the use of intravenous immunoglobulin in the treatment of streptococcal toxic shock syndrome. *Clinics in Infectious Diseases* **26**: 639–641.

40. Arnow PM, Flaherty JP (1997) Fever of unknown origin. *Lancet* **350**: 575–580.

41. Forsyth JRL (1998) Typhoid and paratyphoid. In: *Topley and Wilson's Microbiology and Microbial Infections, vol. 3, Bacterial Infections* (eds Hausler WJ Jr, Sussman M), pp 459–478. Arnold, London.

42. Azad AK, Islam R, Salam MA *et al.* (1997) Comparison of clinical features and pathologic findings in fatal cases of typhoid fever during the initial and later stages of the disease. *American Journal of Tropical Medicine and Hygiene* **56**: 490–493.

43. Mirza SH, Beeching NJ, Hart CA (1996) Multiple drug-resistant typhoid: a global problem. *Journal of Medical Microbiology* **44**: 317–319.

44. Gilbert RJ, Humphrey TJ (1998) Food-borne gastroenteritis. In: *Topley and Wilson's Microbiology and Microbial Infections, vol. 3, Bacterial Infections* (eds Hausler WJ Jr, Sussman M), pp 539–565. Arnold, London.

45. Ramos JM, García-Corbeira P, Aguado JM *et al.* (1996) Classifying extraintestinal non-typhoid *Salmonella* infections. *Quarterly Journal of Medicine* **89**: 123–126.

46. Threlfall EJ, Hall MLM, Rowe B (1992) *Salmonella* bacteraemia in England and Wales, 1981–1990. *Journal of Clinical Pathology* **45**: 35–36.

47. Thamlikitkul V, Dhiraputra C, Paisarnsinsup T et al. (1996) Non-typhoidal Salmonella bacteraemia: clinical features and risk factors. Tropical Medicine and International Health **1**: 443–448.
48. Molyneaux M, Fox R (1993) Diagnosis and treatment of malaria in Britain. British Medical Journal **306**: 1175–1180.
49. Hibbard BM, Anderson MM, Drife JO et al. (1996) Systemic infection. In: Confidential Enquiries into Maternal Deaths in the UK 1991–1993. HMSO, London.
50. Stirrat GM (1994) Pregnancy and immunity. British Medical Journal **308**: 1385–1386.
51. Korzeniowski OK (1995) Antibacterial agents in pregnancy. Infectious Disease Clinics of North America **9**: 639–651.
52. Chernoff AE, Snydman DR (1993) Viral infections in the intensive care unit. New Horizons **1**: 279–301.
53. Read RC (1999) Treating influenza with zanamivir. Lancet **352**: 1872–1873.
54. Cohen JI, Brunell PA, Straus SE et al. (1999) Recent advances in varicella-zoster infection. New England Journal of Medicine **130**: 922–932.
55. Lee WM (1997) Hepatitis B virus infection. Medical progress. New England Journal of Medicine **337**: 1733–1745.
56. Di Bisceglie AM (1998) Hepatitis C – seminar. Lancet **351**: 351–355.
57. Feucht H-H, Schröter M, Zöllner B et al. (1999) Age-dependent acquisition of hepatitis G virus/GB virus C in a non-risk population: detection of the virus by antibody. Journal of Clinical Microbiology **37**: 1294–1297.
58. Winston DJ, Ho WG, Champlin RE (1990) Cytomegalovirus infections after allogeneic bone marrow transplantation. Review of Infectious Diseases **12** (Suppl 7): 776–792.
59. Mocroft A, Youle M, Morcinek J et al. (1997) Survival after diagnosis of AIDS: a prospective observational study of 2625 patients. British Medical Journal **314**: 409–413.
60. BHIVA Guidelines Coordinating Committee (1997) British HIV Association guidelines for antiretroviral treatment of HIV seropositive individuals. Lancet **349**: 1086–1092.
61. Vincent J-V, Anaissie E, Bruining H et al. (1998) Epidemiology, diagnosis and treatment of systemic Candida infection in surgical patients under intensive care. Intensive Care Medicine **24**: 206–216.
62. Rex JH, Rivaldi MG, Pfaller MA (1995) Resistance of Candida species to fluconazole. Antimicrobial Agents and Chemotherapy **39**: 1–8.
63. Burnie JP (1997) Antibiotic treatment of systemic fungal infections. Current Anaesthesia and Critical Care **8**: 180–183.
64. Walsh TJ, Finberg RW, Arndt C et al. (1999) Liposomal amphotericin B for empirical therapy in patients with persistent fever and neutropenia. New England Journal of Medicine **340**: 764–771.
65. Humphreys H, Johnson EM, Warnock DW et al. (1991) An outbreak of aspergillosis in a general ITU. Journal of Hospital Infection **18**: 167–177.

9 Abdominal infections

Infection arising in the peritoneal cavity may be difficult to diagnose in a sedated patient already in the intensive care unit (ICU); therefore a high level of suspicion should be maintained and early investigation undertaken to expedite drainage of infected collections (see Chapters 4 and 5). These infections can be difficult to treat especially if diagnosis is delayed. This chapter discusses acute pancreatitis, peritonitis and intra-abdominal abscess, and urinary and biliary tract infections.

ACUTE PANCREATITIS

Aetiology and incidence

Acute pancreatitis is a relatively common disease with an incidence of 10–20 cases per 100 000 population. Improvement in techniques used to diagnose acute pancreatitis or increasing alcohol abuse in some populations may be factors in the apparent 10-fold increase in incidence over the last 25 years[1, 2]. The two commonest causes are gallstones and alcohol: gallstones in approximately 45% and alcohol in 35%. Ten per cent of cases are idiopathic and the remainder are due to a variety of causes (Table 9.1) including pancreatic or biliary obstruction, trauma, toxins, drugs, infections and metabolic disorders[1].

Pathogenesis

The sequence of events leading from the diverse causes listed above to the activation of trypsin (believed to be an initiating factor) has not been fully elucidated. Trypsinogen is activated to trypsin within the pancreatic acini which, in large amounts, overwhelms naturally occurring inhibitors and triggers the release and activation of an array of cytokines and enzymes including bradykinins, lipases, complement, elastase and phospholipase A_2, and early production of oxygen free radicals[1, 3]. The events that follow range from a mild interstitial inflammation of the pancreas with little systemic upset to widespread pancreatic and peripancreatic necrosis with multiple organ dysfunction, probably associated with bacterial translocation in the later stages[4].

The initial insult to the pancreas causes inflammatory cells to migrate into the interstitium due to upregulation of receptors on polymorphonuclear granulocytes and on endothelium. The inflammatory and clinical features of systemic inflammatory response syndrome (SIRS) mediated by cytokines occur (Chapter 1), and there is some evidence that there is a low serum concentration of the

Table 9.1 Known causes of acute pancreatitis.

Cause	Examples
Obstruction	Gallstones, pancreatic and ampullary tumours
Toxins and drugs	Alcohol, azathioprine, mercaptopurine, frusemide and salicylates
Infection	Mumps, Coxsackie virus, cytomegalovirus and hepatitis A, B and non-A, non-B viruses
Metabolic	Hypertriglyceridaemia and hypercalcaemia
Trauma	Blunt, penetrating and iatrogenic (ERCP)[a]
Miscellaneous	Crohn's disease, duodenal ulcer and vascular abnormalities

[a] ERCP, endoscopic retrograde cholangiopancreatography.

anti-inflammatory cytokine interleukin-10 in severe pancreatitis, suggesting increased consumption not matched by increased production[5].

Presentation and diagnosis

The diagnosis of acute pancreatitis is made by eliciting clinical symptoms and signs together with the use of biochemical and radiographic techniques. Symptoms include upper abdominal pain, back pain and vomiting, and signs vary from mild abdominal tenderness to rebound tenderness, tachycardia and pyrexia. In severe acute pancreatitis, these findings are dramatic, sometimes with flank or periumbilical ecchymoses. Multiple organ dysfunction may also be present as shock evolves.

Leukocytosis is common but not invariably present. Serum amylase concentration is often raised to over 1000 IU, but false-positive results can occur with other causes of an acute abdomen such as a perforated peptic ulcer, and a delay in presentation or the timing of the assay may give a false-negative result. Acute or chronic pancreatitis and alcoholic pancreatitis may not produce such a large rise in serum amylase levels, and increased levels of serum lipase may then be useful[1]. Trypsinogen 2 can be measured in urine as a rapid screening test[6].

Ultrasonography (US) of the biliary tract may indicate the cause and is relatively cheap and accessible. However, dynamic contrast-enhanced computed tomography (CT) produces better images of the pancreas and has been used to determine the severity of pancreatitis and to predict outcome (Figure 9.1, Table 9.2)[7]. Severe acute pancreatitis is defined as pancreatic necrosis of at least 30% of the gland (Plate 9)[8]. CT also identifies many of the other local complications of the disorder (Table 9.3) and is therefore of benefit in the continued management of the very ill patient (see below).

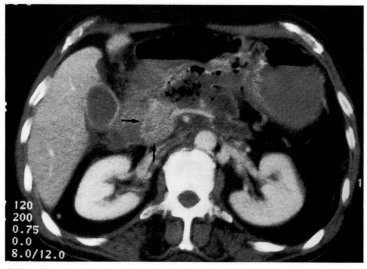

Figure 9.1   CT scan of abdomen demonstrating haemorrhagic necrotizing pancreatitis (arrows).

Table 9.2   Grading of acute pancreatitis using contrast-enhanced CT.

Normal
Focal or diffuse pancreatic oedema
Extension of inflammatory changes into peripancreatic fat
Single ill-defined pancreatic fluid collection
Two or more collections or presence of gas in the pancreas

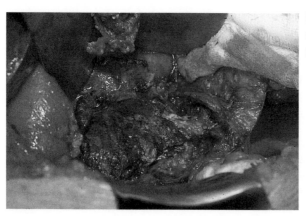

Plate 9   Operative view of necrotizing pancreatitis.

Table 9.3 Complications of acute pancreatitis.

Local
Pancreatic/peripancreatic necrosis ± infection
Acute fluid collection
Pseudocyst
Abscess
Haemorrhage
Bile duct obstruction
Bowel obstruction
Ascites
Hydronephrosis
Gastrointestinal haemorrhage

Systemic
Cardiovascular
  Hypotension
  Shock
  Pericardial effusion
Pulmonary
  Pleural effusion
  Atelectasis
  Pneumonia
  Acute respiratory distress syndrome
Renal
  Oliguria
  Acute tubular necrosis
  Renal artery or vein thrombosis
Haematological
  Disseminated intravascular coagulation
Metabolic
  Hypocalcaemia
  Hyperglycaemia
  Hyperlipidaemia
  Metabolic acidosis
Neurological
  Retinopathy
  Psychosis

Endoscopic retrograde cholangiopancreatography (ERCP) may also be of use to diagnose pancreatitis due to small tumours, gallstones and strictures.

Infective complications

Pancreatic and peripancreatic necrosis, often associated with multiple organ dysfunction, tend to occur in the early stages of acute haemorrhagic pancreatitis[9, 10].

133

Infection of necrotic pancreas occurs in less than 4% of all patients, mainly by translocation of gastrointestinal tract bacteria into the peritoneum, but may also arise via the bloodstream, bile and pancreatic duct[3]. Signs suggestive of infection (e.g. fever, tachycardia and leukocytosis) are often present prior to confirmation of infection in these patients, and therefore any deterioration in clinical condition should arouse suspicion of infected necrotic tissue. *Escherichia coli* is isolated in approximately 30% of cases followed by enterococci in 25%, staphylococci in 15%, *Pseudomonas* spp. in 11% and streptococci in 5%[6]. Monomicrobial infection may later become polymicrobial. Pancreatic necrotic infection occurs during the first, second and third week after presentation in 24, 36 and 71% of cases respectively[11]. This complication is responsible for 70–80% of deaths, although respiratory failure may be a more common cause in the first week[1]. Abscess and pseudocyst formation are typically late complications and intravascular catheter-related sepsis has an increased incidence in these patients of 10–18%[3].

Management

Despite efforts to develop specific therapy, the management of acute pancreatitis continues to rely on the removal of the aetiological factor, supportive therapy and close monitoring for, and the treatment of, complications as they arise. The British Gastroenterological Society has recently issued guidelines and standards for management[12]. Ranson's criteria[13], the Acute Physiology and Chronic Health Evaluation (APACHE) II Score[14] and CT appearances may be used to indicate the severity of acute pancreatitis and predict outcome. Using Ranson's criteria (Table 9.4), patients with one to two risk factors have a mortality rate of less than 1%, those with three to five have a mortality rate of 15%, and patients with six to seven risk factors rarely survive[13]. Serum protein markers (C-reactive protein, complement fractions) can also assess disease severity but have not yet proved to be useful in clinical decision-making[3].

Removal of the aetiological factor

Precipitating drugs or toxins (including alcohol) must be removed. Surgical removal of gallstones in the early stages of the illness is not recommended, but ERCP and sphincterotomy, in experienced hands, may reduce morbidity and mortality.

Supportive therapy

Provision of analgesia and intravenous hydration are mandatory. In patients with ileus or vomiting, nasogastric aspiration may offer symptomatic relief, but has not been shown to reduce hospital stay[1]. Reducing the activity of the pancreas with agents including somatostatin or octreotide, glucagon, atropine and histamine H_2 antagonists has not been associated with any benefit, and enzyme inhibition with aprotinin and gabexate also appears not to offer any advantage[1, 3, 15].

Table 9.4 Ranson's criteria[a].

	Alcoholic pancreatitis	Gallstone pancreatitis
On admission to hospital		
Age	>55 years	>70 years
White cell count	>16 000 mm^{-3}	>18 000 mm^{-3}
Glucose	>11.1 mmol l^{-1}	>12.2 mmol l^{-1}
Lactate dehydrogenase	>350 units l^{-1}	>400 units l^{-1}
Aspartate aminotransferase	>250 units l^{-1}	>250 units l^{-1}
Within 48 hours of admission		
Decrease in haematocrit	>10 points	>10 points
Increase in blood urea nitrogen	>1.79 mmol l^{-1}	>0.71 mmol l^{-1}
Serum calcium	<2 mmol l^{-1}	<2 mmol l^{-1}
Arterial oxygen pressure	<60 mmHg	Not applicable
Base deficit	>4 mmol l^{-1}	>5 mmol l^{-1}
Estimated fluid deficit	>6 liters	>4 liters

[a] Each of the values of variables listed constitutes a risk factor; the number of risk factors determines prognosis. See text for mortality rates associated with number of risk factors.

Treatment of organ dysfunction

Cardiovascular instability may require large volumes of intravenous fluids to replace transcapillary losses, and inotropes and/or vasoactive agents. These should be guided by appropriate invasive monitoring such as pulmonary arterial catheterization. Serum electrolytes, in particular calcium, magnesium and potassium, should be maintained within the normal range. Respiratory failure may be due to abdominal 'splinting', basal atelectasis, pleural effusions, fluid overload or non-cardiogenic pulmonary oedema. Renal dysfunction may necessitate the use of a renal replacement therapy such as continuous venovenous haemofiltration.

Treatment of infective complications

Prolonged peritoneal lavage for a period of 7 days in patients with severe pancreatitis may reduce pancreatic abscess formation but has not shown any beneficial effect on mortality[16]. Subtotal pancreatectomy has a mortality rate of 33% and most survivors develop diabetes mellitus. Surgery remains the treatment of choice for infected pancreatic necrosis and the drainage of infected fluid collections. There is controversy as to whether sterile necrosis should be surgically debrided or treated conservatively, as recovery of a patient with pancreatic necrosis is not uncommon, providing infection does not occur[3, 17, 18]. CT-guided fine-needle aspiration followed by immediate culture of necrotic material should be performed to differentiate sterile from infected necrosis. Iatrogenic infection during the procedure is rare[19]. Drainage of acute fluid collections may also be possible by CT guidance although 50% of these resolve spontaneously. Pseudocysts and abscesses usually require at least 4 weeks to develop and can often be drained percutaneously under CT guidance. However, many pseudocysts resolve spontaneously in patients with minimal symptoms.

There seems to be no indication for other surgical intervention; a recent study from France showed no improvement in mortality by debridement, closed lavage, enteral (jejunostomy) feeding and loop ileostomy to prevent the complication of colonic ischaemia[16]. ERCP and sphincterotomy within 24 hours may reduce mortality in patients with pancreatitis due to gallstones[20, 21]. Gallstone pancreatitis will require elective (interval) cholecystectomy after the patient is fully recovered.

Role of antibiotics

Bacterial infection occurs in 40–70% of patients and contributes to mortality. Since there is a close correlation between infection and outcome in severe acute pancreatitis, antibiotic prophylaxis has been suggested by some trials[22]. Early studies used antibiotics subsequently shown to have poor pancreatic penetration. Imipenem and quinolones, however, penetrate pancreatic tissue well, whereas aminoglycosides do not. Metronidazole and clindamycin also achieve reliable therapeutic tissue levels. One recent study with imipenem prophylaxis showed a reduction in pancreatic sepsis although overall mortality was unaffected[23], whereas another study in which cefuroxime was administered did show a reduction in mortality[24]. Some clinicians therefore use prophylactic antibiotics in those patients with severe disease or with acute pancreatic necrosis on CT, and a combination of a quinolone (e.g. ciprofloxacin, i.v., 400 mg 12-hourly) and metronidazole (500 mg 8-hourly), or a cephalosporin antibiotic are appropriate choices. Selective decontamination of the digestive tract (SDD) reduces the number of pancreatic infections but has not yet been shown to reduce mortality, although those with severe disease may benefit slightly. Recent evidence regarding use of SDD suggests that this approach may be of some benefit generally in the ICU patient but it remains debatable as to whether it should be routine for this group of patients[25]. Finally, there is some preliminary evidence in favour of a platelet-activating factor (PAF) antagonist, lexipafant, in reducing the incidence of organ failure associated with infection[26].

Nutrition

Severe pancreatitis has been considered an absolute contraindication to enteral feeding in order to rest the gut but this is based on the belief that the necrotic gland is still secreting activated enzymes. Enteral feeding at the jejunal level, however, does not stimulate the pancreas as long as medium-chain triglycerides provide fat requirements. Studies have compared total parenteral nutrition (TPN) with no nutrition and found no difference in outcome but more rapid resolution of pancreatitis and shorter hospital stay were observed in the unfed group[27]. There are now reports of the beneficial use of enteral nutrition, probably best delivered distal to the ligament of Treitz, where cholecystokinin is secreted into the third part of the duodenum, as jejunal delivery of feed is not associated with an increase in pancreatic exocrine secretory volume, or secretion of protein or bicarbonate. A randomized study of enteral versus parenteral feeding in acute pancreatitis, in which a semi-elemental enteral feed was used, demonstrated that there were fewer septic complications and no adverse effects in those patients receiving enteral feeding[28].

Outcome

The overall mortality rate in acute pancreatitis is approximately 9% but may be reduced in the severe form of illness by tertiary referral[29]. Mortality is related to certain risk factors as illustrated by the use of Ranson's criteria (Table 9.4). The mortality rate can be as high as 60% when infection of pancreatic or peripancreatic necrosis occurs, compared with 5.9% in patients with sterile necrosis. Organ failure is the most important determinant of death.

PERITONITIS AND INTRA-ABDOMINAL ABSCESS

Aetiology

Perforation of the gastrointestinal tract is the most common cause of intra-abdominal infection. Intestinal ischaemia, anastomotic leak and abdominal trauma account for most of the remainder. Intra-abdominal infection presents either as secondary peritonitis due to one of the causes referred to above or as a discrete abscess[30]. Primary peritonitis, usually monobacterial, occurs when ascites becomes infected without visceral disruption and is nowadays seen most commonly in patients undergoing continuous ambulatory peritoneal dialysis (CAPD). Persistent peritoneal infection in critically ill patients caused by resistant or unusual organisms is an increasing challenge.

Pathogenesis

When organisms from the gastrointestinal tract gain access to the peritoneal cavity, they are rapidly swept towards the diaphragm and absorbed by the lymphatics, sometimes giving rise to bacteraemia, and about 40% of these patients will develop shock. However, if conditions are present that hinder this clearance (e.g. necrotic tissue), or the initial bacterial load is very large, organisms may persist in the peritoneal cavity. Phagocytosis by macrophages then occurs and these cells are slowly replaced by polymorphonuclear leukocytes as time evolves. The greater omentum can prevent spread of bacteria but, if infection persists, abscess formation may occur. In addition to these host defence mechanisms, fibrin may seal perforations and limit bacterial spread but may also hinder antimicrobial and phagocytic cell penetration. Capillary permeability increases during this process which may lead to hypovolaemia, with fluid collecting in the peritoneal cavity and the bowel.

Most patients with secondary peritonitis have polymicrobial infection. *Bacteroides fragilis* is the anaerobe most often isolated, with *E. coli* the commonest aerobe. *Pseudomonas* spp. are recovered in a small minority. However, a study of severely ill patients operated on with culture-proven intra-abdominal infections and a preoperative APACHE II score greater than or equal to 15 reported a different spectrum of organisms. *Candida* spp. were isolated in 41%, enterococci in 31%, *Enterobacter* spp. in 21%, *Staphylococcus epidermidis* in 21%, streptococci in 17% and *E. coli* in only 17%. Almost two-thirds of patients had polymicrobial infections. The authors concluded that intra-abdominal infections in critically ill patients were often due to different organisms than those found in less severely ill patients[31]. Persistent peritonitis in ICU patients also shows this pattern; fungi were isolated in 72%, *S. epidermidis* in 64%, *Pseudomonas* spp. in 48%, *Enterobacter* spp. and enterococci each in 32%, *E. coli* in 24% and *B. fragilis* in only 12% in one particular study[32]. Selective antibiotic pressure, gut mucosal damage, multiple abdominal surgery and malnutrition are probable risk factors for *Candida* infection and infection with resistant bacteria.

Presentation and diagnosis

Following contamination of the peritoneal cavity, there is often an initial peritonitis and bacteraemia due to Gram-negative aerobes. The abscess formation seen at a later stage is more commonly due to anaerobes. Patients with peritonitis usually present with a 'hyperdynamic' circulation, but sometimes bacteraemia or remote organ failure may be due to intra-abdominal infection without diagnostic abdominal signs. Plain X-ray of the abdomen may confirm visceral perforation when free gas is present, and may also show a gas–fluid interface in an abscess, or organ displacement (Figure 9.2).

Ultrasonography has a high sensitivity (60–90%) for detecting abscesses and its accessibility, lack of ionizing radiation and cost-effectiveness are advantageous, but interloop abscesses are not well demonstrated and bowel gas, lung and skin surface obstructions are major limitations. CT is superior to US for demonstrating abscesses in all areas of the abdomen except perhaps the pelvis, and has a sensitivity greater than 90%. It has become the investigation of choice for confirming intra-abdominal fluid collections. The sensitivity of both US and CT is reduced in the postoperative period due to irrigation, oedema, blood in the peritoneum and ileus, and therefore false-negative examinations may occur[33].

Management

The objectives are to eliminate the source of the peritoneal contamination, remove any fluid collections, provide appropriate supportive care and eliminate residual contamination with antimicrobial agents.

Supportive therapy

Respiratory and cardiovascular support may be required, particularly during the bacteraemic phase. Hypovolaemia is common and invasive monitoring is often required to prevent underestimation of fluid requirements.

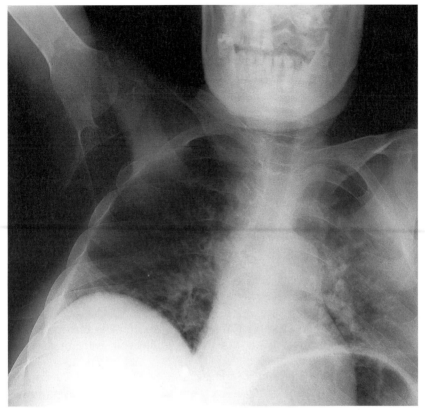

Figure 9.2 Plain erect abdominal X-ray showing visceral perforation; florid example of air under diaphragm.

Surgery and peritoneal decontamination

Surgery is required to close perforations, remove necrotic bowel and flush out peritoneal contamination. Postoperative lavage does not improve outcome, although planned relaparotomy at 12–48-hour intervals may be of value in patients with severe diffuse peritonitis and multiple organ dysfunction[31]. Open management (laparostomy) aids re-exploration and can reduce high intra-abdominal pressure. Percutaneous drainage of established abscesses under US or CT is often possible and has a similar outcome as surgical drainage[13], but is less successful when abscesses are loculated, multiple or poorly organized. Fungal abscesses, infected haematomas and necrotic tissue cannot, however, be treated by percutaneous drainage. In general, small and deep collections are more easily located by CT[33].

Antibiotic therapy

Anaerobic and aerobic Gram-negative organisms must be covered when treating secondary peritonitis but the optimum duration of treatment remains a matter of opinion. Metronidazole (i.v., 500 mg 8-hourly) is the first-line treatment for anaerobic intra-abdominal infection, but in the USA clindamycin (600–1200 mg 6-hourly) is preferred. The combination of an expanded-spectrum cephalosporin (e.g. cefotaxime, i.v., 1–2 g 8-hourly) and an aminoglycoside (e.g. gentamicin, i.v., 5 mg kg^{-1} once daily) is recommended for the treatment of aerobic Gram-negative bacillary infections. Despite the fact that aminoglycosides are less active at the low pH found in peritoneal infection, these agents retain a place in therapy as resistance to them is still low in many centres and they are rapidly bactericidal. Once-daily dosing is supported by theoretical and animal studies and minimizes toxicity, but studies on critically ill humans (with altered pharmacokinetics) are limited[31]. Bacteria that produce β-lactamases (e.g. *Enterobacter* spp., *Pseudomonas* spp., *Serratia* spp., *Providencia* spp. and *Acinetobacter* spp.) may be resistant to cephalosporins and therefore alternative antimicrobial agents such as a quinolone (e.g. ciprofloxacin, i.v., 400 mg 12-hourly) should be considered. The combination of an antipseudomonal penicillin with a β-lactamase inhibitor (e.g. piperacillin–tazabactam, i.v., 4.5 g 8-hourly) broadens the spectrum of activity to cover anaerobes, but *Enterobacter* spp., *Serratia* spp. and *Pseudomonas* spp. other than *P. aeruginosa* may be resistant[31]. The carbapenems (meropenem, 1 g 8-hourly, and imipenem, 500–1000 mg 6-hourly) have good activity against aerobic Gram-negative bacilli and anaerobes but are often reserved for second-line therapy. However, overuse of carbapenems gives rise to superinfection with multi-resistant *Stenotrophomonas maltophilia*.

The isolation of enterococci in complicated intra-abdominal infection may predict failure of treatment[34]. However, there is at present controversy over the benefits of using specific therapy against *Enterococcus* spp. in intra-abdominal infections as these organisms may only be a cofactor for *B. fragilis* infection. Nevertheless, severe infections associated with enterococcal bacteraemia or a predominance of enterococci in peritoneal fluid culture should be treated. Ampicillin (1 g 6-hourly), perhaps combined with an aminoglycoside (e.g. gentamicin, 5 mg kg^{-1} once daily), is the agent of choice. Vancomycin (i.v., 1 g 12-hourly) or teicoplanin are also effective against enterococci but the emergence of vancomycin-resistant enterococci (VRE) in some centres limits its use. It is essential that regular monitoring of aminoglycoside and vancomycin blood levels takes place in these critically ill patients takes place to ensure optimal therapy and to minimize toxicity.

The assessment and treatment of *Candida* intra-abdominal infections is difficult. *Candida* may be cultured from peritoneal fluid in stable patients but if there is associated candidaemia then antifungal therapy should commence. Histological evidence of invasive candidal infection from surgical specimens also indicates the need for specific therapy, as does a failure of response to appropriate antibacterial drugs in critically ill patients. Amphotericin B (i.v., up to 1.5 mg kg^{-1} day^{-1}) is the most effective antifungal agent but is nephrotoxic, although liposomal formulations (e.g. AmBisome, i.v., 3 mg kg^{-1} day^{-1}) are less toxic but expensive[35]. Both agents require a test dose before the administration of the full dose due to the risk of anaphylaxis. Fluconazole (i.v., 400 mg day^{-1}) is an alternative but its inactivity against some *Candida* strains limits its usefulness in critically ill patients. This is also discussed in Chapter 8.

Outcome

This is related to the source of infection, the severity of the systemic response, the patient's premorbid physiological reserve and the speed and appropriateness of early management. Peritonitis due to appendicitis or perforation of a duodenal ulcer has a mortality rate of 1–20%. Peritonitis due to other perforations is associated with a mortality rate of 20–50%, and postoperative peritonitis has a mortality rate of 40–60%. The mortality rate due to intra-abdominal infection increases by 20–30% when complicated by bacteraemia. When acute renal failure occurs the mortality rate is 40–70% and if the acute respiratory distress syndrome develops the rate can be as high as 85%[31].

URINARY TRACT INFECTION (UTI)

Aetiology

Bacterial pathogens causing nosocomial UTI usually originate from the patient's faecal flora; *E. coli* is responsible for approximately 50% (up to 90% of community-acquired infections), *Klebsiella* spp. for 15–20%, *P. aeruginosa* for 10–15%, enterococci for 10–12% and *Proteus* spp. for 10–12%. Less commonly, *Enterobacter* spp. *Citrobacter* spp., *Acinetobacter* spp., *Serratia* spp., *Staphylococcus aureus* and coagulase-negative staphylococci cause UTI[36]. In critically ill patients, *Candida* spp. are also an important cause of UTI and may be the first sign of a systemic fungal infection. They are more common in catheterized patients and those receiving antibacterial agents.

Pathogenesis

Bacteraemia may sometimes cause a UTI by seeding in the kidney, e.g. a renal abscess due to *S. aureus*. More commonly, predisposing factors for an ascending UTI include instrumentation of the urinary tract (including catheterization) and obstruction to urinary flow. Instrumentation is implicated in approximately 80% of nosocomial UTIs[37]. Critically ill patients require precise urine flow measurement and will therefore be catheterized, and at increased risk of UTI. Micro-organisms can reach the bladder either via the lumen of the catheter (although this is rare if a closed drainage system is in use), or by ascending between the wall of the catheter and the mucous membrane of the urethra. Once this occurs, the development of infection depends on a balance between the bacterial growth rate and the urinary flow. The latter is often reduced in critically ill patients, adding to the risk of infection. Conditions that favour bacterial growth include a pH between 6.0 and 7.0, and the presence of glucose in the urine.

Incidence

Of patients who undergo urinary catheterization, up to 30% develop significant bacteriuria depending on the technique of insertion and the patient population. Bacteraemia due to catherization occurs in approximately 8%, and up to half of these may develop a clinically significant bacteraemia[37]. The European Prevalence of Infection in Intensive Care Study reported the incidence of urinary tract infection in ICUs as 17.6%, second only to pneumonia and lower respiratory tract infections[36]. However, few patients with UTI alone will require ICU care.

Presentation and diagnosis

Kidney and ureteric infections classically present with fever, rigors and loin pain and may require admission to a high-dependency area; blood and urine should be taken for culture. More commonly, nosocomial infection in critically ill patients is less florid and comprehensive investigation must include urine culture in addition to blood and other specimens if the source is unknown. Urine specimens for culture should be taken by aseptic aspiration of the catheter (not from the catheter bag) and transported to the laboratory as soon as possible. If there is a delay they should be refrigerated at 4°C.

Once the bladder has been catheterized, colonization of the bladder with organisms usually follows in 7–10 days. Traditionally a bacterial count of 100 000 colony forming units (CFU) ml^{-1} has been used to differentiate significant bacteriuria from probable contamination, and polymicrobial infection is considered to indicate contamination. Similarly, *Candida* colony counts above 10^3–10^4 CFU ml^{-1} suggest a UTI although the presence of *Candida* in urine is never considered normal[38]; it may be due to contamination from vaginitis or balanitis and therefore of less clinical significance. These guidelines are not infallible, particularly in catheterized patients. Low colony count bacteriuria (10^2–10^4 CFU ml^{-1}) commonly progresses to high colony counts ($>10^4$ CFU ml^{-1}) within 24–48 hours. The Centers for Disease Control (CDC) have developed a specific definition for nosocomial urinary tract infection[39].

Imaging of the urinary tract may occasionally prove useful in the diagnosis and treatment of UTI, e.g. ultrasonography may indicate an abnormal kidney or an adjacent soft tissue fluid collection.

Management

Prevention of UTI in the ICU is of prime importance. General measures include using a sterile technique for insertion of catheters, maintenance of a closed drainage system, avoidance of contamination by good practice, non-invasive methods of urine collection and hand washing by all staff between patients. More specific preventive measures include antiseptics inserted *per urethra* prior to catheterization and meatally, or into the bladder during the course of catheterization and bladder irrigation with sterile saline in those patients with accretions or blood clots, but these measures have not been proven effective in good clinical trials. Prophylactic antimicrobials may be indicated for instrumentation of the urinary tract of patients with significant bacteriuria but should not be used routinely.

In patients presenting with signs and symptoms of systemic infection in the ICU, treatment is usually required before the results of cultures become available. Empirical treatment should cover the majority of organisms mentioned above. A combination of a penicillin or cephalosporin (e.g. cefotaxime, i.v., 1 g 8-hourly) and gentamicin (i.v., 5 mg kg^{-1} once daily) is usually effective but concerns about renal toxicity may preclude the latter; serum levels should be monitored. In patients with renal impairment, a quinolone (e.g. ciprofloxacin, 200–400 mg 12-hourly) may be used but the dose or dose interval may need to be altered depending on the severity of renal impairment. Duration of antimicrobial treatment should be 5 days although this should be extended in patients with pyelonephritis, to avoid reinfection.

Candidal infection may indicate systemic candidiasis and systemic amphotericin B (i.v., up to 1.5 mg kg^{-1} day^{-1}) is the agent of choice. Treatment of *Candida* UTI confined to the lower urinary tract with amphotericin B bladder washouts (50 mg l^{-1} in sterile water by continuous irrigation or intermittent infusion for 5–7 days) is recommended, although efficacy and toxicity have not been fully evaluated. Fluconazole (400 mg day^{-1} administered systemically) is also effective in the treatment of *Candida* UTI without systemic involvement and is less toxic than parenteral amphotericin B[40].

BILIARY TRACT INFECTION

Any patient in the ICU for a prolonged period is at risk of developing acute cholecystitis, which is difficult to diagnose, and therefore may be life-threatening. Biliary stasis, vascular insufficiency of the gall bladder and toxic factors may all be involved and the major aetiological factor remains contentious, but it is likely that a combination of factors is responsible[41].

Aetiology

The liver acts as a bacteriological filter of the portal tract removing organisms from the circulation into the reticuloendothelial system via the Kupffer cells; it does not secrete bacteria into the biliary system and therefore the biliary tract is usually sterile. However, 30–90% of patients with biliary disease have positive bile cultures. Upper gastrointestinal tract flora such as *E. coli*, enterococci, *Klebsiella* spp. and *Proteus* spp. are the commonest causes of biliary infection. *Enterobacter* spp., *Pseudomonas* spp. and anaerobic bacteria (*Clostridium* spp., *Bacteroides* spp.) are much less commonly isolated, but may be associated with polymicrobial infection and multiple biliary procedures[42]. It should be remembered also that not all cases of cholecystitis are associated with gall-stones, i.e. acalculous cholecystitis.

Pathogenesis

Colonization of the biliary tract is common if the sphincter of Oddi is incompetent or bypassed by sphincterotomy, intestinal anastomosis or the presence of biliary drains. Despite such colonization, patients usually show signs of infection only if biliary drainage becomes obstructed or if gallstones are present. The biliary tract may also become infected if gastrointestinal tract organisms are translocated via the portal vein, such as occurs in patients with obstructive jaundice.

Presentation and diagnosis

In critically ill patients, biliary infection may present acutely as suppurative cholangitis, infective biliary peritonitis or, rarely, gangrenous cholecystitis. A preceding history of biliary tract obstruction is common and high fever, rigors, jaundice and localized or generalized peritonitis may be present. Patients may also present with, or develop, subhepatic or subphrenic abscesses.

Management

Gangrenous cholecystitis or perforation require urgent surgical resection and repair and in patients with cholangitis the obstructed biliary tree must be adequately drained. Increasingly, endoscopic drainage techniques are favoured over a traditional surgical approach as morbidity and mortality may be less. Conservative management with antibiotic therapy and organ support is often successful in the absence of biliary obstruction.

Although it was originally believed that the biliary secretion of antimicrobial agents resulting in high local levels was of prime importance in determining efficacy in biliary tract infection, current opinion is that adequate serum levels of antibiotics predict a successful outcome. In critically ill patients, an extended-spectrum cephalosporin such as cefotaxime (i.v., 1–2 g 8-hourly) should be administered together with metronidazole (i.v., 500 mg 8-hourly). Alternatively, a penicillin–β-lactamase inhibitor combination (such as co-amoxiclav, i.v., 1.2 g 6-hourly, or piperacillin–tazobactam, i.v., 4.5 g 8-hourly) can be used, although the latter may best be reserved as a second-line option[42]. Comparison of drug levels in serum and bile suggests an active secretion of piperacillin and elimination into bile[43] but when the biliary tract becomes obstructed ciprofloxacin, not piperacillin, is actively excreted into bile[44].

Key points

- The two commonest causes of acute pancreatitis are gallstones (45%) and alcohol (35%).
- Grading and assessing the severity of acute pancreatitis is best done using contrast-enhanced CT.
- Reducing the activity of the pancreas with agents such as somatostatin or octreotide, glucagon, atropine and histamine H_2 antagonists has not been shown to be beneficial.
- The mortality rate from acute pancreatitis can be as high as 60% when pancreatic or peripancreatic infection occurs, compared with 5.9% in patients with sterile necrosis.
- Perforation of the gastrointestinal tract is the most common cause of intra-abdominal infection. Intestinal ischaemia, anastomotic leak and abdominal trauma account for most of the remainder.
- The incidence of urinary tract infection in intensive care units is approximately 17.6%.
- Any patient in the ICU for a period of time is at risk of developing acute cholecystitis, which is often difficult to diagnose, and therefore may be life-threatening.

REFERENCES

1. Steinberg W, Tenner S (1994) Acute pancreatitis. *New England Journal of Medicine* **330**: 1198–1210.
2. Thomson SR, Hendry WS, McFarlane GA *et al.* (1987) Epidemiology and outcome of acute pancreatitis. *British Journal of Surgery* **74**: 398–401.
3. Ranson JHC (1982) Etiological and prognostic factors in human acute pancreatitis: a review. *American Journal of Gastroenterology* **77**: 633–638.
4. Lemaire LCJM, van Lanschot JJB, Stoutenbeek CP *et al.* (1997) Bacterial translocation in multiple organ failure: cause or epiphenomenon still unproven. *British Journal of Surgery* **84**: 1340–1350.
5. Pezzilli R, Billi P, Miniero R *et al.* (1997) Serum interleukin-10 in human acute pancreatitis. *Digestive Diseases and Sciences* **42**: 1469–1472.
6. Kemppainen EA, Hedstrom JI, Puolakkainen PA *et al.* (1997) Rapid measurement of urinary trypsinogen-2 as a screening test for acute pancreatitis. *New England Journal of Medicine* **336**: 1788–1793.
7. Kemppainen EA, Sainio V, Haapianen R *et al.* (1996) Early localisation of necrosis by contrast-enhanced computed tomography can predict outcome in severe acute pancreatitis. *British Journal of Surgery* **83**: 924–929.
8. Frileux P, Berger A (1993) Acute pancreatitis: infection, measurement of severity and treatment. *Current Opinion in Surgical Infections* **1**: 89–98.
9. Isenmann R, Buchler M, Uhl W *et al.* (1993) Pancreatic necrosis: an early finding in severe acute pancreatitis. *Pancreas* **8**: 358–361.

10. Tenner S, Sica G, Hughes M et al. (1997) Relationship of necrosis to organ failure in severe acute pancreatitis. *Gastroenterology* **113**: 899–904.
11. Beger HG, Bittner R, Block S et al. (1986) Bacterial contamination of pancreatic necrosis. A prospective clinical study. *Gastroenterology* **91**: 433–438.
12. United Kingdom guidelines for the management of acute pancreatitis. (1998) *Gut* **42** (Suppl 2): S1–S12.
13. Ranson JHC, Rifkind KM, Roses DF et al. (1974) Prognostic signs and the role of operative management in acute pancreatitis. *Surgery, Gynecology and Obstetrics* **139**: 69–81.
14. Larvin M, McMahon MJ (1989) APACHE II score for assessment and monitoring of acute pancreatitis. *Lancet* **ii**: 201–205.
15. McKay C, Baxter J, Imrie C (1997) A randomised, controlled trial of octreotide in the management of patients with acute pancreatitis. *International Journal of Pancreatology* **21**: 13–19.
16. Borie D, Frileux P, Levy E et al. (1994) Surgery of acute necrotizing pancreatitis. Active prolonged drainage in 157 consecutive patients. *Presse Medicale* **23**: 1064–1068.
17. Ranson JHC (1995) The current management of acute pancreatitis. *Advances in Surgery* **28**: 93–112.
18. McFadden DW, Reber HA (1994) Indications for surgery in severe acute pancreatitis. *International Journal of Pancreatology* **15**: 83–90.
19. Balthazar EJ, Freeny PC, van Sonnenberg E (1994) Imaging and intervention in acute pancreatitis. *Radiology* **193**: 297–306.
20. Neoptolemos JP, Carr-Locke DL, London NJ et al. (1988) Controlled trial of urgent endoscopic retrograde cholangiopancreatography and endoscopic sphincterotomy versus conservative treatment for acute pancreatitis due to gallstones. *Lancet* **ii**: 979–983.
21. Fan ST, Lai ECS, Mok FPT et al. (1993) Early treatment of acute biliary pancreatitis by endoscopic papillotomy. *New England Journal of Medicine* **328**: 228–232.
22. Sainio V, Kemppainen P, Puolakkainen P et al. (1995) Early antibiotic treatment in acute necrotising pancreatitis. *Lancet* **346**: 663–667.
23. Perderzoli P, Bassi C, Vesentini S et al. (1993) A randomized multicentre clinical trial of antibiotic prophylaxis of septic complications in acute necrotizing pancreatitis with imipenem. *Surgery, Gynecology and Obstetrics* **176**: 480–483.
24. Barie PS (1996) A critical review of antibiotic prophylaxis in severe acute pancreatitis. *American Journal of Surgery* **172** (Suppl 6A): 38S–43S.
25. D'Amico R, Pifferi S, Leonetti C et al. (1998) Effectiveness of antibiotic prophylaxis in critically ill adult patients: systematic review of randomised controlled trials. *British Medical Journal* **316**: 1275–1285.
26. Kingsnorth AN, for the British Pancreatitis Study Group (1997) Early treatment with lexipafant, a platelet-activating factor antagonist, reduces mortality in acute pancreatitis: a double-blind, randomized placebo controlled study (Abstract). *Gastroenterology* **112** (Suppl): A453.
27. Sax HC, Warner BW, Talamini MA et al. (1987) Early total parenteral nutrition in acute pancreatitis: lack of beneficial effects. *American Journal of Surgery* **153**: 117–124.
28. Kalfarentzos F, Kehagias J, Mead N et al. (1997) Enteral nutrition is superior to parenteral nutrition in severe acute pancreatitis: results of a randomized prospective trial. *British Journal of Surgery* **84**: 1665–1669.

29. Malcynski JT, Iwanow IC, Burchard KW (1996) Severe pancreatitis. Determinants of mortality in a tertiary referral centre. *Archives of Surgery* **131**: 242–246.

30. McClean KL, Sheehan GJ, Harding GKM (1994) Intraabdominal infection: a review. *Clinical Infectious Diseases* **19**: 100–116.

31. Sawyer RG, Rosenlof LK, Adams RB *et al.* (1993) Peritonitis into the 1990s: changing pathogens and changing strategies in the critically ill. *American Surgeon* **58**: 82–87.

32. Rotstein OD, Pruett TL, Simmons RL (1986) Microbiological features and treatment of persistent peritonitis in patients in the intensive care unit. *Canadian Journal of Surgery* **29**: 247–250.

33. Montgomery RS, Wilson SE (1996) Intraabdominal abscesses: image-guided diagnosis and therapy. *Clinical Infectious Diseases* **23**: 28–36.

34. Burnett RJ, Haverstock DC, Dellinger EP *et al.* (1995) Definition of the role of *Enterococcus* in intraabdominal infection: analysis of a prospective randomized trial. *Surgery* **118**: 716–723.

35. Tang CM, Bowler ICJW (1997) Do the new lipid formulations of amphotericin B really work? *Clinical Microbiology and Infection* **3**: 283–288.

36. Vincent JL, Bihari DJ, Suter PM *et al.* (1995) The prevalence of nosocomial infection in intensive care units in Europe; results of the European Prevalence of Infection in Intensive Care (EPIC) Study. *Journal of the American Medical Association* **274**: 639–644.

37. Meares EM (1991) Current patterns in nosocomial urinary tract infections. *Urology* **37** (Suppl 3): 9–12.

38. Stamm WE (1991) Catheter-associated urinary tract infections: epidemiology, pathogenesis, and prevention. *American Journal of Medicine* **91** (Suppl 3B): 65S–71S.

39. Garner JS, Jarvis WR, Emori TG *et al.* (1988) CDC definitions for nosocomial infections, 1988. *American Journal of Infection Control* **16**: 128–140.

40. Voss A, Meis JFGM, Hoogkamp-Korstanje JAA (1994) Fluconazole in the management of fungal urinary tract infections. *Infection* **4**: 247–251.

41. Boland G, Lee MJ, Mueller PR (1993) Acute cholecystitis in the intensive care unit. *New Horizons* **1**: 246–260.

42. van den Hazel SJ, Speelman P, Tytgat GNJ *et al.* (1994) Role of antibiotics in the treatment and prevention of acute and recurrent cholangitis. *Clinical Infectious Diseases* **19**: 279–286.

43. Westphal JF, Brogard JM, Caro-Sampara F *et al.* (1997) Assessment of biliary excretion of piperacillin–tazobactam in humans. *Antimicrobial Agents and Chemotherapy* **41**: 1636–1640.

44. van den Hazel SJ, de Vries XH, Speelman P *et al.* (1996) Biliary excretion of ciprofloxacin and piperacillin in the obstructed biliary tract. *Antimicrobial Agents and Chemotherapy* **40**: 2658–2660.

10 Multiple trauma and soft tissue infections

MULTIPLE TRAUMA

Patients with multiple trauma represent a significant proportion of admissions to intensive care units (ICUs), especially units located near busy motorways and major road systems. Of 10 000 patients surveyed in the European Prevalence of Infection in Intensive Care (EPIC) Study, 13% were admitted with multiple trauma and, after final statistical analysis, trauma on admission was found to be an independent risk factor for unit-acquired infection[1]. The successful management of the patient with multiple trauma is dependent on an understanding of the pathophysiological changes that take place, constant review and assessment of all organ systems and multidisciplinary involvement in diagnosis and treatment. Whilst infection is not usually of major concern during the initial stabilization process, measures adopted then to improve oxygen delivery and organ blood flow may subsequently help to minimize the risk of infection and multi-organ failure (MOF) and are therefore of great importance (Chapter 6). Close collaboration between intensivists, surgeons, radiologists and microbiologists/infectious disease physicians and ICU nurses is essential to ensure optimal care.

The systemic effects of multiple trauma

Severe injury evokes a systemic response from cells of the immune system resulting in the secretion of cytokines and other metabolic products which result in many beneficial but also some deleterious effects on various organ systems. It is believed that an initial massive traumatic insult can create a severe systemic inflammatory response syndrome (SIRS) independent of infection (one-hit model). Alternatively, a less severe traumatic insult can create an inflammatory environment (i.e. primes the host) such that later an otherwise innocuous, secondary inflammatory insult precipitates severe SIRS (two-hit model).

When natural and acquired immunity are disturbed as occurs following serious injury, increased susceptibility to infection follows. This impaired immunity is characterized by diminished production of interleukin 2 (IL-2) and T helper (T_H) lymphocytes. Exposure of naive T_H cells to certain antigens and cytokines causes conversion to either the T_H1 or the T_H2 phenotype. T_H1 cells produce IL-2 and interferon γ and initiate cellular immunity. T_H2 cells secrete IL-4 and IL-10 and stimulate production of certain antibodies. Conversion to the T_H1 and T_H2 phenotypes is facilitated by IL-2 and IL-4, respectively. Massive complement activation may also occur and may contribute to MOF. Removal of the activated complement components from the circulation is difficult, however, as much of the protein is attached to cell membranes, hence inhibition of the enzymatic cascade may be more appropriate (see Chapters 1 and 6). These patho-physiological changes ultimately result in a SIRS that also occurs in infection, burns, pancreatitis and after major surgery (see Chapter 1).

The major initial challenge is to maintain physiological stability during resuscitation, especially when attempting to control haemorrhage, or in the management of injury itself, to mitigate the effects of metabolic acidosis, hypothermia and coagulopathy; the lethal triad of death[2]. Early deaths are related to uncontrolled haemorrhage, the severity of injury and development of brainstem death. Shock and the subsequent reperfusion injury that occurs after resuscitation initiates a sequence of events leading to progressive cellular dysfunction throughout the body that ultimately contributes to MOF[3]. Free oxygen radicals are formed during reperfusion and measures to scavenge them, such as intravenous mannitol or vitamins C and E, or to block xanthine oxidase, may improve outcome[4, 5]. In haemodynamically unstable trauma patients, failure to restore the splanchnic circulation as demonstrated by gastric intra-mucosal pH <7.32 results in both an increased incidence of MOF and risk of death[6].

Hypothermia due to heat loss in the field (e.g. at the roadside following a major traffic accident) or during resuscitation, or arising from exposure of body cavities during surgery and from transfusion of inadequately warmed blood, is another factor influencing outcome. Adverse effects of hypothermia include[7]:

1. Cardiac arrhythmias
2. Reduced cardiac output
3. Increased systemic vascular resistance
4. Immunosuppression
5. Coagulopathy leading to disseminated intravascular coagulation.

Early management

The initial management of the patient with multiple trauma should follow advanced trauma life support (ATLS) guidelines which involve stabilization of cardiac and respiratory function. Full investigation of injuries and prioritization of surgical repair should follow and this may include exploratory laparotomy for control of haemorrhage and contamination, evacuation of intracranial haematomas or insertion of transducers to monitor intracranial pressure. Early stabilization of fractures is usually undertaken but depends on the stability of the patient. Initial laparotomy may involve simple vascular repairs, stapling or suturing of hollow viscus injuries, defunctioning ostomies with thorough wash-out and rapid closure of the abdomen. Open fractures that are associated with arterial injuries must be managed immediately if amputation is to be avoided[8]. The next stage in the resuscitation process will usually take place in the ICU and requires involvement of a full critical care team to oversee haemodynamic stabilization, core rewarming, the restoration of intravascular volume and ventilation. This secondary resuscitation period, which may take up to 48 hours, also influences outcome and unplanned reoperations such as to control bleeding will adversely affect outcome.

The abdominal compartment syndrome illustrates very well many of the above physiological changes associated with multiple trauma. It is characterized by massive abdominal distension and multi-system dysfunction including decreased cardiac output due to preload reduction and vena caval obstruction. The measurement of intravesical pressure may be useful in diagnosis. Reduced perfusion of the gastrointestinal tract occurs resulting in mucosal acidosis and impaired barrier function, impaired jugular drainage and raised intracranial pressure, reduced diaphragmatic excursion and raised pleural pressure[9]. Successful management incorporates abdominal decompression with the restoration of intravascular volume and organ support.

Ongoing intensive care

After 12–24 hours the life-threatening effects of major trauma, such as multiple open fractures, lacerations to the spleen and liver, and intracranial haemorrhage, will have been identified and in most cases stabilized. However, a full head-to-toe inspection is required, if it has not already been carried out, to identify other injuries not immediately apparent and to detect early infection. This should be repeated especially if the patient's condition becomes unstable. Planned reoperation may be required, either to follow up the initial exploratory laparotomy or to carry out a definitive procedure. There is no ideal time for this, but within 36 hours following admission to the ICU after organ function is stabilized is preferred. Reoperation will usually involve irrigation and careful exploration to search for missing injuries, ligation of bleeding vessels, removal of devitalized tissue and, depending upon the injuries, the insertion of a feeding jejunostomy tube[10]. Where a patient returns to theatre for further management of open fractures, the wound should be carefully examined circumferentially and covered but not sutured.

Repeated debridement every 48–72 hours may be necessary to establish a viable environment for soft tissue coverage[8]. Then, good-quality microbiological specimens, such as tissue, fluid or pus, rather than swabs, can be obtained to guide subsequent antibiotic use. It is important to indicate clearly where and when the sample was obtained to avoid confusion later or when interpreting the significance or otherwise of a positive growth. Apart from ICU-acquired infection, bacteraemia or lower respiratory tract infections, major wound infections due to serious degloving injuries or following early closure of the abdomen under tension are a significant risk. A high index of suspicion should be maintained for the presence of intra-abdominal infection in the pyrexial patient and abscess formation should be sought aggressively and drained under ultrasonography. Computed tomography (CT) and magnetic resonance imaging (MRI) may be more sensitive but are often not possible in the unstable patient. Colonic injuries require very careful resuscitation and exploration with close postoperative monitoring for septic complications. The risk of intra-abdominal infection, including secondary peritonitis, is increased after multiple procedures and spillage from hollow viscera, and may occur in approximately half of cases[10].

INFECTIVE COMPLICATIONS OF TRAUMA

The nature of the infective complication will depend on the severity and extent of trauma and any other underlying disease present, such as chronic lung disease. Wound infection and osteomyelitis (not always apparent for some time afterwards) are the main direct infective complications.

The skin forms an important part of the innate defences against topical and other infections. Exposed dry areas such as the arms support the growth of relatively few organisms due to the dryness and relatively high salt content of this environment. Moist areas such as the perineum support the growth of a greater number and variety of organisms and this is one of the main reasons why the femoral area is not a good site for intravascular catheter insertion. The microbiological flora of the skin can be subdivided into resident and transient flora. The resident flora of the normal skin, including the sebaceous and sweat gland follicles, consists predominantly of *Staphylococcus epidermidis*, micrococci, diphtheroids and some anaerobic cocci. These are relatively avirulent microbes except in the presence of prosthetic material such as intravascular catheters, or in the severely immunocompromised patient. The transient flora of the skin, however, is more varied and may be acquired from the environment, heavily colonized areas such as the gastrointestinal tract or other people. Transient flora consists of *Staphylococcus aureus*, enterobacteria such as *Escherichia coli*, and *Candida* spp., but under normal circumstances the intact skin, fatty acids on the skin itself and washing limit the survival and growth of such organisms. The presence of denuded areas of skin such as may follow burns or wounds (surgical or traumatic) provides the opportunity for these microbes to survive and thrive, and furthermore they can easily be transmitted via the hands of health care workers, especially in the absence of good hand-washing practice.

Wound infections
Pathogenesis and aetiology
Following trauma, wound infection may arise from deep lacerations and compound fractures, and the source of infection may be the patient's own flora, bacteria from other patients (i.e. cross-infection) or organisms acquired from the environment, e.g. soil at a road traffic accident site. For example, a penetrating stab wound to the abdomen may become contaminated with spores of *Clostridium tetani* (see Chapter 11). The physiological condition of the wound is also important as tissue necrosis, vascular strangulation, haematoma, excessive oedema, poor blood supply and poor oxygenation all compromise the normal defence mechanisms. The risk of wound infection is also higher in the elderly, obese patients, patients with diabetes mellitus and those on immuno-suppressive medications. Burns and areas of tissue necrosis are susceptible to infection with *S. aureus* but other bacteria such as β-haemolytic streptococci and *Bacteroides* spp. may also be implicated.

Pseudomonas aeruginosa may cause severe infections in burns patients with loss of skin grafts, bacteraemia and septic shock. However, in the majority of instances, *P. aeruginosa* like many other Gram-negative bacilli colonizes rather than infects wounds. Gas gangrene (see below) caused by *Clostridium perfringens* may develop rapidly (i.e. within hours) following trauma and subsequent MOF is due to the production of numerous exotoxins leading to tissue damage and muscle death. Necrotizing fasciitis (see below) may develop after penetrating injuries, major burns and even surgical procedures. The superantigen effects of streptococcal toxins activate many cells of the immune system leading to overwhelming inflammation[11]. Wounds arising from dog or cat bites, although not a common reason for admission to the ICU, may be associated with an adverse outcome if the wounds are extensive, the patient debilitated, or serious infection ensues. As well as staphylococcal, streptococcal and anerobic organisms, infections from dog or cat bites are commonly caused by *Pasteurella* spp., the most common isolate recovered in a recent series[12]. These bacteria as well as *Capnocytophaga canimorsus*, which is also associated with animal bites, may result in systemic infection, including bacteraemia and gangrene, especially in the immunocompromised patient such as the diabetic. Tetanus is also a theoretical complication and should be considered in management (see below).

Presentation

Gross contamination of the wound may not always be apparent at the time of trauma, or subsequently, but there is a higher risk of infection following surgery for a perforated viscus. Untreated, dirty wounds are especially likely to become infected as clinically apparent by the presence of erythema and pus. Wounds should therefore be inspected regularly in all patients following multiple trauma.

Management

Aggressive surgical debridement to remove necrotic and potentially infected tissue is the key to a good outcome. Tissue rather than swabs should be sent to the microbiology laboratory for culture and sensitivity as this will help guide subsequent antibiotic therapy if required (see below). Generally, major traumatic wounds should be left unsutured and high-dose benzylpenicillin (e.g. i.v., 1.2–1.8 g 4–6-hourly) given to minimize the risk of gas gangrene. In patients with compound fractures, prophylaxis with a cephalosporin such as cefuroxime (i.v., 1.5 g) is advised and regular review of all traumatic wounds is essential. Tetanus immunization should also be reviewed (see Chapter 11) and a dose of tetanus immunoglobulin (i.m., 250–500 IU) administered, if more than 24 hours have elapsed since the injury or there is a risk of heavy contamination or following burns[13].

Osteomyelitis
Pathogenesis and aetiology

Unlike childhood osteomyelitis, which is usually haematogenous, bone infection in adults is often associated with trauma, or occurs following local or contiguous infection, or following the insertion of a foreign body such as an orthopaedic pin or screw. Whilst superficial skin or wound infection may be present shortly after trauma, osteomyelitis may not be diagnosed for some weeks or even months later. Once infection has become established, pus spreads into the vascular channels, raising the intraosseous pressure and impairing blood flow, which in turn compromises local immune defences. The aetiological organisms are more varied than those causing haematogenous infection, e.g. *S. aureus* is not so common; coliforms such as *E. coli*, and *Klebsiella* spp. and anaerobes may all be implicated, and polymicrobial infection is not uncommon.

Diagnosis

Clinical assessment and a variety of imaging techniques such as CT or MRI will confirm the diagnosis, but surgical sampling or a needle biopsy of infected tissue provides the indispensable information to permit the identification of the causative organism and to guide appropriate antimicrobial therapy[14]. Superficial swabs or sampling of the fluid exiting from sinuses often merely reflect local skin flora rather than the causative pathogen.

Management

Parenteral antibiotic administration for at least 4 weeks before extensive destruction of bone has occurred is recommended to achieve an acceptable cure rate[14]. Because of the limited bioavailability of high-dose oral β-lactam antibiotics, such as flucloxacillin or cefuroxime, and poor gastrointestinal tolerance, early intravenous–oral switch therapy is not advisable in adults with acute osteomyelitis. Whilst long-term oral therapy with quinolones such as ciprofloxacin may suppress and occasionally eradicate infection where the pathogen is susceptible, there is a significant risk of resistance emerging especially if used as single-agent therapy. The choice of agent will depend on the aetiology. Staphylococcal infection may be treated with flucloxacillin (i.v., 1–2 g 6-hourly) or with fusidic acid (orally, 500 mg 8-hourly); fusidic acid penetrates bone tissue well and oral administration is associated with a lower risk of cholestatic jaundice than parenteral administration. Gram-negative infection may be treated with a combination of an extended-spectrum cephalosporin (e.g. ceftazidime, i.v., 2 g 8-hourly) or a quinolone (e.g. ciprofloxacin, i.v., 400 mg 12-hourly) or with an aminoglycoside such as gentamicin, $5 \, mg \, kg^{-1} \, day^{-1}$ (amikacin may be indicated for gentamicin-resistant pathogens). However, gentamicin blood levels should be monitored regularly to minimize toxicity and to optimize therapy but expert advice should be sought on the basis of the microbiological culture and antibiotic susceptibility results.

Eye infections
Pathogenesis and aetiology

Eye infections are relatively unusual under normal circumstances because of the eyelids, ocular secretions and a variety of non-specific immune defence mechanisms. However, in the comatose patient, inability to shut the eyes, inadequate blinking and intermittent positive pressure ventilation, which encourages body fluid retention, predispose to bacterial keratitis[15] and even ophthalmitis. Apart from *S. aureus* and other pyogenic bacteria such as the pneumococcus, Gram-negative bacteria including *P. aeruginosa* are implicated[16]. However, it can sometimes be difficult to distinguish colonization from infection and a specialist opinion from an ophthalmologist should be sought if necessary.

Presentation and diagnosis

Ocular erythema and discharge are characteristic of keratitis but endophthalmitis may be suggested by corneal oedema or ulcers, and orbital cellulitis[16]. Where efforts are made to confirm a diagnosis microbiologically, the majority of specimens are positive, especially if vitreous fluid is sent for culture.

Management and outcome

Antibiotics to treat eye infections may be given by the topical, subconjunctival, intraocular or systemic routes but difficulties in penetrating to the eye chambers should ensure that the treatment of serious keratitis or endophthalmitis be left to the specialist. The fluoroquinolones, such as ciprofloxacin, are increasingly effective whereas the cephalosporins and macrolides are less useful due to significant pharmacokinetic shortcomings[17]. As approximately 60% of patients with culture-positive endophthalmitis may lose vision in the affected eye, especially if caused by *P. aeruginosa*, prevention is critical. Measures to reduce the incidence of both keratitis and endophthalmitis include avoiding multi-use ointment tube or drop applicators in more than one patient, not applying patches to eyes with discharge, not leaving contact lenses *in situ*, avoiding routine eye swabs, which are not necessary, and not suctioning respiratory tract secretions across the head of the patient without covering the eyes[15].

THE USE OF ANTIBIOTICS IN THE MANAGEMENT OF MULTIPLE TRAUMA

Prophylaxis

Whilst the judicious use of antibiotics is important in minimizing the occurrence of infection and in controlling infection when it does occur, antibiotics alone are no substitute for appropriate surgical care and resuscitation, including the removal and/or drainage of infected material. The use of prophylactic antibiotics in trauma differs somewhat from routine surgical prophylaxis, e.g. to cover elective large bowel resection. In patients with multiple trauma, antibiotics are often continued for somewhat longer periods to cover the immediate resuscitation period and beyond, despite a paucity of evidence to justify more than one or two doses. When a patient has one or more open fractures, especially if severe or involving the lower leg with soft tissue damage, prophylaxis is strongly recommended[8, 18]. Open fractures of the lower leg with overlying tissue damage result in infection in as many as 50% of patients. A first- or second-generation cephalosporin such as cefuroxime (i.v., 1.5 g) is usually adequate unless the patient has recently received antibiotics, or is at particular risk of infection with resistant organisms. Antibiotics should normally be given for only 24 hours.

Spinal procedures associated with trauma, especially those involving insertion of metal rods, require prophylaxis. There is no indication for prophylactic anti-biotics following skull fracture or cerebrospinal fluid (CSF) leaks but patients should be monitored closely for signs and symptoms of meningitis. Patients requiring neurosurgical procedures require a second-generation cephalosporin for clean, non-implant procedures and co-amoxiclav for clean-contaminated procedures (see Chapter 11)[19].

Prophylaxis is also indicated following penetrating abdominal injuries and should be continued for 12–24 hours if bowel perforation is confirmed, but in most other circumstances a single dose of an antibiotic should suffice[20]. Whichever antibiotics are chosen for prophylaxis, they should be safe, effective against the bacteria most likely to cause infection and likely to achieve high concentrations in the tissues most at risk of becoming infected. Antibiotic resistance is not usually a major concern when choosing the antimicrobial agent as patients with multiple trauma are likely to become infected in the first instance with community-acquired pathogens, which are usually fairly sensitive, unless there has been a period of recent hospitalization. It is only later, when infection is fully established or acquired in the ICU, that the local antibiotic resistance pattern of local flora will influence the choice of agent(s) for treat-ment. Furthermore, the emergence of resistance is minimal if prophylaxis is confined to one to three doses. A cephalosporin, with metronidazole if anaerobic bacteria are likely to be implicated, is generally appropriate. Suggested antibiotic regimens and duration of prophylaxis are indicated in Table 10.1.

Selective decontamination of the digestive tract (SDD)

SDD consists of use of topical antibiotics (e.g. tobramycin, polymyxin and amphotericin B) applied to the oral mucosa and given through the nasogastric tube throughout the ICU admission, with parenteral antibiotics such as an extended-spectrum cephalosporin for the first 3–4 days. This approach has been advocated to reduce the incidence of nosocomial infection in patients with multiple trauma because it is believed that it preserves the protective effects of endogenous flora, especially anaerobic bacteria, and prevents colonization or infection with potential pathogens such as S. aureus, enterococci, Klebsiella aerogenes, P. aeruginosa and Candida spp. Early studies in patients with multiple trauma and other patients admitted to the ICU demonstrated reduced colonization with potential pathogens and a significant reduction in ICU-acquired infection[21,22]. Other studies confirmed a reduction in ventilator-associated pneumonia and a decrease in the overall cost of antimicrobial agents in patients with multiple trauma but no effect on overall mortality[23]. The absence of an obvious impact on mortality, concerns over the possible emergence of multiple antibiotic resistance in these patients on prophylactic antibiotics for long periods of time, and the perception that SDD significantly increases intensive care costs, have discouraged many from using this approach routinely.

Table 10.1 Options for prophylactic antibiotics in patients with multiple trauma.

Category of injury	Recommendations
Abdominal	Cefuroxime, i.v., 1.5 g plus metronidazole, i.v., 500 mg once Three doses if perforated viscus
Orthopaedic	Benzylpenicillin, i.v., 600 mg for 5 days, to prevent gas gangrene following amputations or major surgery associated with significant contamination Cephradine, i.v., 1 g or cefuroxime, i.v., 1.5 g, one to three doses for open fractures

Head and neck
  Head injuries/CSF leaks
  Maxillofacial trauma
	No prophylaxis
	Co-amoxiclav, i.v., 1.25 g, three doses

Urological and vascular	No prophylaxis required unless significant contamination or special circumstances, then co-amoxiclav, i.v., 1.25 g, one to three doses

Nonetheless, a recent meta-analysis of randomized controlled trials has demonstrated a reduction in respiratory infection from 36% amongst controls to 16% in patients receiving SDD and suggests that maximum efficiency is achieved when both topical and systemic antibiotics are used[24]. The effect of this intervention in terms of the number of patients needing treatment to prevent one infection and one death is significant, however, at 5 and 23 patients respectively, but compares favourably with many other interventions in clinical practice[24]. Each ICU therefore needs to review its patient profile in terms of the reason for admission, the incidence of ICU-acquired infection, potential cost savings and the local antibiotic resistance patterns when making a decision as to whether to use SDD on all or selected patients such as those following multiple trauma.

Therapeutic antibiotic use

It is important to reassess the choice of antibiotics if infection becomes established or arises subsequently during or following prophylaxis. In general, it is wise to use different antibiotics for prophylaxis and for treatment. Consequently, extended-spectrum cephalosporins such as cefotaxime and ceftazidime, fluoroquinolones such as ciprofloxacin, piperacillin–tazobactam and meropenem should not be used prophylactically unless significant antibiotic resistance is prevalent in the ICU or the individual patient is known to be colonized with bacteria susceptible only to these second-line agents. Restricting the use of these agents for specific patients has the further benefit of helping to contain ICU drug costs. Combination antimicrobial chemotherapy may be required initially pending the results of culture or to treat polymicrobial infection. For example, intra-abdominal infection caused by aerobic and anaerobic bacteria may be treated initially with gentamicin, cefotaxime or ciprofloxacin, with metronidazole. More specific therapy, e.g. flucloxacillin for confirmed methicillin-sensitive staphylococcal infection, is indicated following microbiological confirmation and the results of susceptibility testing (see Chapter 5 for further details).

Infection prevention in the asplenic patient

Life-threatening infection is now well recognized as a major long-term risk following splenectomy, i.e. overwhelming post-splenectomy infection (OPSI), as splenic macrophages have an important filtering and phagocytic role in removing bacteria from the circulation. Every effort should be made to retain the intact spleen or part thereof in order to maintain immune function but where this is not possible, due to severe damage or major haemorrhage, consideration must be given to minimizing the long-term complications. The organisms most likely to cause serious infection are outlined in Table 10.2.

A working party of the British Committee for Standards in Haematology has produced consensus recommendations for managing patients without a spleen[25]. Most infections occur within the first few years of splenectomy when the consequent mortality rate is higher. All patients following splenectomy, or those who are autosplenectomized such as patients with sickle cell disease after splenic infarcts or those with bone marrow transplants or patients receiving immunosuppressive therapy, should receive *Haemophilus influenzae* type b vaccine owing to the risk of OPSI. The polyvalent pneumococcal polysaccharide vaccine is recommended for any patient over 2 years of age with asplenia or severe dysfunction of the spleen (except those who are pregnant).

Table 10.2   Organisms causing life-threatening infection following splenectomy.

Encapsulated bacteria
Streptococcus pneumoniae
Haemophilus influenzae type b
Neiserria meningitidis

Other organisms
E. coli
C. canimorsus[a]
Plasmodium (malaria)
Babesia (babesiosis)

[a] Associated with bacteraemia following dog bite.

Ideally, vaccination to prevent these infections should be administered before splenectomy to maximize protection (see also chapter 5). Clearly this is not possible when splenectomy is associated with multiple trauma but should be given at least 2 weeks before elective splenectomy when at all possible. It is therefore important to ensure that all patients who have undergone splenectomy do not leave the ICU or hospital before appropriate vaccinations and antibiotics have been organized. Immunization should be delayed for 6 months after immunosuppressive therapy, during which time prophylactic antibiotics must be given. The following vaccines should be given[25]:

1. Pneumococcal vaccine: this is 90% effective in healthy adults under the age of 55 years but revaccination is recommended every 5–10 years.
2. *Haemophilus* vaccine type b: most patients over 18 years of age will have acquired some immunity but this may not provide adequate protection for patients with an absent or dysfunctional spleen.
3. Meningococcal vaccine: there is currently no vaccine against the most common strains causing disease in temperate climates, i.e. group B strains, but those patients travelling to areas of the world where other strains are more common, e.g. group A in the Middle East, should be vaccinated accordingly. Group C vaccination may become routine shortly.
4. Influenza vaccine reduces the incidence of infection with this underestimated pathogen and any secondary bacterial infection that may follow.

Further details on the dosage regimens, methods of administration, the need for boosters and possible side-effects can be found elsewhere[13].

Long-term antibiotic prophylaxis is another measure that helps to reduce life-threatening infection following splenectomy. Whilst it is likely that many patients may not be highly motivated to take drugs indefinitely for a potential risk of infection when they are otherwise well, prophylactic antibiotics should be offered in all cases, and strongly recommended especially in the first 2 years after splenectomy. Oral penicillin (500 mg twice daily) is appropriate, or erythromycin (250 mg twice daily) in the penicillin-allergic patient. Finally, the patient (when they are well enough), their close relatives and their general practitioner should be fully informed of the risk of infection, especially OPSI. Patients should be strongly advised to consult their doctor early if they develop an infection and they should also be warned about the need for precautions against mosquito and tick bites when travelling abroad to minimize the acquisition of tropical diseases such as malaria. Asplenic patients should wear a Medi-Alert disc or equivalent to alert paramedics and accident and emergency staff to their vulnerability to OPSI.

INFECTION AND BURN INJURIES

Aetiology

Host immunity becomes depressed 7 days after burn injury and the degree of immunosuppression is correlated with the size of the burn. Both humoral and

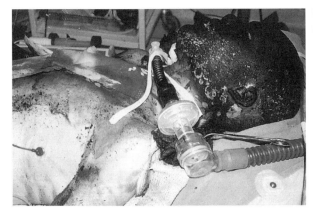

Plate 10 Extensive burns with fasciotomy.

cell-mediated immunity are affected as are reticuloendothelial and phagocytic function. Gram-positive, Gram-negative, fungal and viral organisms can therefore all cause infection in these patients. In addition, translocation of intestinal bacteria into the portal circulation, and nosocomial pneumonia (particularly in intubated patients following inhalational thermal injury), are additional infective risks in patients who have suffered burn injuries. Where burn injuries are greater than 40% of the skin surface, the high mortality rate is attributed primarily to infection, most commonly pneumonia, burn wound infection and septicaemia (Plate 10).

Pathogenesis
Colonizing bacteria, normally or transiently resident on the skin surface (e.g. *S. aureus*, Gram-negative bacilli), are able to invade once the skin barrier is breached by the burn and host defences are sometimes unable to prevent spread to adjacent tissues. Tissue necrosis and exudate subsequently encourage bacterial proliferation. Systemic spread is also possible but bacteraemia is less common than the symptoms and signs might suggest. Gram-positive organisms initially predominate in burn wounds, but later become replaced by Gram-negative organisms including *Pseudomonas* spp. *Proteus* spp. and *Klebsiella* spp., and *Candida albicans*.

Diagnosis
Burn injury infection and sepsis may be difficult to diagnose because an inflammatory response is an integral part of the host response to the burns. Blood cultures are frequently sterile and wound cultures may only reflect colonization. Constant surveillance is required to diagnose systemic infection.

Management
Supportive care
Respiratory distress must be treated promptly with supplemental oxygen and, if necessary, with tracheal intubation and with mechanical ventilation. Upper airway

burns may produce laryngeal oedema and airway obstruction making intubation hazardous, and an inhalational induction with intubation under deep volatile anaesthesia must be considered in all cases. Smoke inhalational injury is suggested by burns in and around the airway and by carbonaceous sputum. Carbon monoxide levels may be high and carboxyhaemoglobin levels must be measured.

Assessment of burn wound area and thickness allows calculation of estimated fluid replacement but deviation from standard formulae may be required according to the clinical situation; invasive monitoring of the central venous pressure is useful to guide fluid replacement. A nasogastric tube should be passed in all patients with major burns to prevent gastric distension.

All burns should be gently cleaned and devitalized tissue removed. Early debridement with skin grafting has recently become the management of choice for full (and perhaps partial) thickness burns as this reduces the risk of infective complications[26]. When enough skin cannot be harvested to cover all the wound, repeated procedures at weekly intervals will be required. Cadaveric and synthetic skin may be used as temporary wound cover.

Metabolism increases dramatically after a burn injury, reaching twice normal when the burn area is 60% of body surface area, and results in net catabolism with breakdown of muscle protein for energy production[27]. This is partly due to the endotoxaemia that often occurs as a result of loss of integrity of the mucosal layer of the intestine and early enteral feeding should be commenced to attempt to prevent this. SDD (see above) appears to reduce the infective complications and mortality of burn injury[27–29], but this is not standard practice in many centres.

Infection prevention and antibiotics

Good practice, especially compliance with hand-washing protocols, is paramount to reducing secondary infection in patients with extensive burn injuries. Ideally, patients should be isolated in rooms with positive pressure ventilation. Mupirocin, applied to the nostrils three times daily for 5 days, reduces the carriage of S. aureus but the increasing prevalence of resistant strains, especially methicillin-resistant S. aureus (MRSA), suggests that this useful topical agent should be used more carefully.

Prophylactic systemic antibiotics are not recommended; they do not penetrate burn injuries reliably and may encourage development of resistant organisms, e.g. MRSA, and C. albicans. However, bacteraemia during surgical interventions is common, and antibiotic therapy should be considered. If systemic infection is thought likely, parenteral empirical therapy with a combination of benzylpenicillin (1.2–1.8 g 4–6-hourly), flucloxacillin (1 g 6-hourly) and gentamicin (5 mg kg^{-1} once daily) with measurement of serum levels is appropriate.

Topical agents delay wound colonization and reduce wound flora. Silver sulfadiazine 1% is most commonly used[26] but may delay keratinocyte proliferation and therefore early skin grafting is the treatment of choice[27]. When silver sulfadiazine is used, it should be reapplied every 24–48 hours. Leukopenia may occur shortly after the commencement of silver sulfadiazine treatment but this does not lead to an increased infective risk and cell counts usually recover spontaneously in spite of continued usage.

Outcome

Improvements in management, including early debridement and perhaps early enteral nutrition, have led to an increased survival in the best centres. Sixty years ago, the mean burn area associated with a 50% survival rate was 30% of body surface area; now there is a 50% mortality rate from a 65–75% burn[27].

DEGLOVING INJURIES

If digits or limbs are trapped during injury the skin and subcutaneous tissue are ripped off the underlying tissue. It is important that these injuries are properly treated. The skin should not be rolled back as this predisposes to infection but subcutaneous fat should be removed and a skin graft applied. These injuries are best managed by plastic surgeons but it is essential that all contaminated tissue and foreign material are removed.

SOFT TISSUE INFECTIONS

Necrotizing fasciitis
Aetiology

This is an uncommon subcutaneous tissue and superficial fascia infection that is associated with systemic toxicity, a fulminant course and a high mortality rate. Bacterial growth is present in the vast majority of appropriate specimens sent for culture and mixed aerobic/anaerobic bacteria are recovered from the majority. The predominant aerobes include *S. aureus*, *E. coli* and group A streptococci (often associated with this condition on its own) and the predominant anaerobes are *Peptostreptococcus* spp., *Prevotella* spp. and *Prophyromonas* spp.[30]. *Vibrio vulnificus*, an organism normally found in sea water, is also associated with necrotizing fasciitis in certain countries and exposure to shellfish is associated with infection due to this bacterium[11]. Anaerobic organisms associated with large bowel flora play a major role in the aetiology of the related Fournier's gangrene and necrotizing cellulitis (see below). Despite effective antibiotics and the use of intravenous immunoglobulin the mortality rate from this condition has not decreased and remains at about 35%[31].

Pathogenesis

Necrotizing fasciitis usually follows trauma and results in gangrene of the skin due to rapid spread of toxin-producing bacteria along ischaemic or avascular tissue planes within the subcutaneous soft tissues (Figure 10.1). It occurs most commonly in the elderly, diabetics and those with impaired defence mechanisms,

161

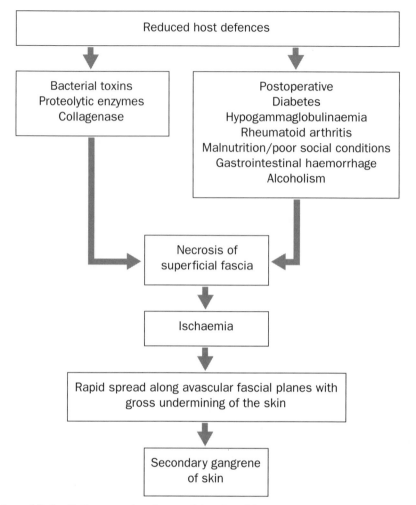

Figure 10.1 Pathogenesis of necrotizing fasciitis.

e.g. alcoholics, patients on steroids and parenteral drug abusers. It has also been suggested that the presence of chickenpox and use of non-steroidal anti-inflammatory drugs may be predisposing factors[11]. The streptococcal exotoxins (superantigens) have the ability to stimulate the immune system and produce a cascade of cytokines responsible for inducing toxic shock (Chapter 8)[32, 33]. Streptolysin O can also induce production of tumour necrosis factor.

Presentation
Eighty per cent of patients have a history of minor trauma such as a cut or insect bite (often not remembered by the patient), minor burn or surgical

incision and, occasionally, ischiorectal abscess, abdominal surgery or fractured pelvis are the initiating events. Scrotal infection is called Fournier's gangrene and this may spread rapidly to the perineum and abdominal wall. The limbs (particularly lower) are the most common sites of necrotizing fasciitis. The area infected becomes shiny, erythematous and very tender, dusky areas appear within the cellulitic areas and haemorrhagic bullae may occur. Skin ulceration reveals underlying gangrene, and gas may be present. By now there is often less pain in the affected area, but toxaemia is pronounced and spread of the necrosis is alarmingly rapid due to immunological features resulting in an Arthus or Schwartzmann reaction and the release of bacterial enzymes such as hyaluronidase or fibrinolysin. Necrotizing cellulitis is a variant of necrotizing fasciitis where skin and muscle are also affected.

Diagnosis

Diagnosis is difficult during the early stages and involves differentiation from gas gangrene (muscle involvement), cellulitis (less systemic toxaemia) and myositis (muscle involvement with minimal skin changes). Cultures from several sites should if possible be taken early (pus or tissue samples rather than swabs); blood cultures should be taken but are usually sterile as toxaemia rather than bacteraemia is characteristic. Gram stain of tissues may be useful but often reveals many different organisms. Microscopic examination of frozen-section material taken at the time of surgical debridement can be useful.

Management

Fluid resuscitation with invasive monitoring, early aggressive surgery to remove necrotic tissue and to provide samples to confirm the diagnosis, and broad-spectrum intravenous antibiotics (until the results of culture and antibiotic susceptibility tests are available) are the principles of effective management. Correction of disseminated coagulopathy with blood products may also be required.

Radical excisional surgery or debridement improves survival, albeit at the cost of greater final deformity[34]. Debridement should extend into normal healthy fascia and the wound should be left open to permit regular reinspection. Ideally tissue should be taken before any antibiotics are given but often parenteral antibiotics have already been started empirically. A preferred initial combination might be high-dose cefotaxime (2 g 8-hourly), metronidazole (500 mg 8-hourly) and gentamicin (5 mg kg^{-1} daily; serum levels should be monitored). Subsequent therapy will depend upon the result of Gram staining and cultures. Benzylpenicillin (i.v., 1.2–1.8 g 4–6-hourly) is still the drug of choice in sensitive monomicrobial streptococcal infection but clindamycin (i.v., 600–1200 mg 6-hourly) should be considered as an alternative for patients with established invasive infection, because this drug inhibits the metabolic activity of the streptococcus and production of toxins. Antibiotic-associated diarrhoea due to *Clostridium difficile*, however, is a major complication of clindamycin use but it must be remembered that about one-third of patients admitted to the ICU will develop diarrhoea due to medication or enteral feeding as well as due to antibiotic therapy[35]. The use of hyperbaric oxygen to supplement antibiotics is still advocated for patients with Fournier's gangrene[36], but is associated with some logistical problems. Human immune globulin contains toxin-neutralizing antibodies and, if given at an early stage of invasive disease, may be of benefit[37].

Outcome
The mortality rate is 20–50% and early recognition and aggressive treatment are paramount in improving the prognosis of this condition.

Gas gangrene
Aetiology
Necrosis of muscle due to toxigenic clostridial infection is the characteristic feature of gas gangrene. These bacteria are Gram-positive, spore-forming, obligate anaerobes that are widely present in soil and normal colonic flora. Commonest amongst those causing gas gangrene is *C. perfringens*, although polymicrobial infection is very common. *C. novyi*, *C. septicum* and *C. histolyticum*[38], other non-toxigenic clostridia and facultative aerobes, e.g. *E. coli* and *Proteus* spp., may also be present. The aerobes assist in promoting ideal conditions for clostridial growth by utilizing oxygen for their metabolism.

Pathogenesis
Trauma to tissues leads to contamination if these organisms are present in the local environment (soil, weapons or endogenous bowel flora present on the skin or clothing). Postoperative wound contamination may occur, as may myometrial contamination during abortion or (rarely) childbirth. Wound contamination is eradicated by cleaning and innate defence mechanisms usually prevent infection. However, clostridial cellulitis occurs in circumstances similar to that of necrotizing fasciitis if surrounding tissue is damaged, foreign material is present, where there is poorly perfused or necrotic tissue, and if the host immune system is impaired, with diabetic patients being particularly at risk (Figure 10.1). Necrosis impairs the function of phagocytic cells as they are unable to gain access to areas of infection. Infection spreads slowly to adjacent areas involving local fascial planes with mild muscle inflammation, although systemic toxaemia can be significant. Later, invasion of healthy muscle by micro-organisms following toxin-induced necrosis leads to further myonecrosis and systemic toxaemia (gas gangrene). Toxin formation by clostridia is central to the disease progression. *C. perfringens* produces a number of toxins; α toxin (a phospholipase) is associated with capillary and blood cell damage and, in synergy with other bacteria, damages surrounding tissue thus accelerating bacterial spread. Collagenase, hyaluronidase, fibrinolysin and deoxyribonuclease are also produced by *C. perfringens* and contribute to tissue necrosis.

Acute renal failure, hypotension, jaundice and altered cerebral state are systemic sequelae of clostridial infection and an enhanced awareness by the patient of their surroundings, progression to a toxic confusional state, and finally coma, are characteristic clinical features.

Incidence

Traumatic wounds and postsurgical wounds account for most cases of gas gangrene outside war-torn areas. Up to 80% of traumatic open wounds may be contaminated by clostridia, but gas gangrene is a rare infection, even in battlefield injuries. In the developed world, the incidence amongst the civilian population is believed to be 0.1–1 per 10^6 of the population per year[38].

Presentation

Clostridial cellulitis presents with skin and underlying subcutaneous erythema. Inflammation associated with a wound but without systemic upset is usual in the early stages. Gas may be present and, due to minimal oedema, may be easily detected early. As fascial planes become involved, the syndrome progresses rapidly and systemic toxaemia then develops. Pain, oedema, haemorrhagic exudate within bullae and tachycardia all suggest the development of gas gangrene, although the presence of gas may not be as obvious as in clostridial cellulitis. Myometrial infection is not common except following septic abortion when abdominal pain and a haemorrhagic cervical discharge are specific features.

Diagnosis

Diagnosis is primarily based on clinical features as the isolation of clostridia from wounds does not automatically indicate disease due to the ubiquitous nature of these bacteria. Alternative diagnoses to be considered are fasciitis and necrotizing cellulitis.

Haemolytic anaemia, thrombocytopenia and coagulation defects occur during clostridial sepsis. Plain X-rays of the affected area may demonstrate gas in the affected tissues (Figure 10.2), although this appearance may be produced by other bacteria.

Gram stain of a specimen of wound exudate will demonstrate Gram-positive rods, and clostridia may be isolated in 18–24 hours. During surgery, affected muscle is oedematous and non-contractile when stimulated by surgical instruments; a frozen section of affected muscle may confirm the diagnosis.

Management

Surgery to remove necrosis and reduce the bacterial load is essential in cases of spreading infection and myonecrosis, and where signs of systemic sepsis are present. Amputation, hysterectomy or excision of other affected tissues is urgently required, and must extend into healthy tissue to ensure adequate clearance. Repeated wound inspections and, if necessary, further debridement in theatre must be performed regularly.

Benzylpenicillin in large doses (i.v., 2.4 g 4–6-hourly in adults) is the antibiotic of choice. Metronidazole, together with cefotaxime (i.v., 2 g 8-hourly), is an alternative if other bacteria are implicated or in patients with penicillin allergy.

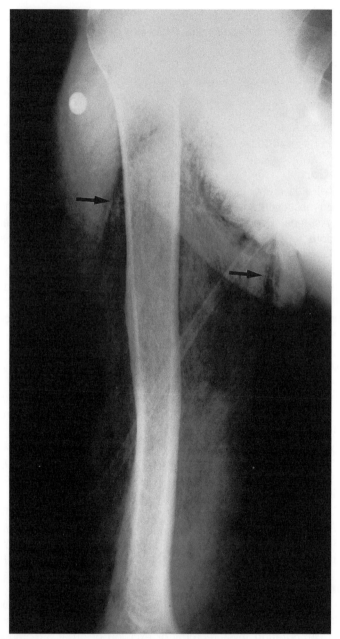

Figure 10.2 Gas in the subcutaneous tissues (arrows) surrounding the humerus, characteristic of gas gangrene.

Hyperbaric oxygen therapy has been reported to improve the prognosis from gas gangrene in combination with the above measures, on the basis of experimental and clinical evidence rather than from clinical trials. Transporting critically ill patients is a significant risk, and therefore should be considered only if it is available locally. Treatment consists of oxygen at 1.5–2 atmospheres for about 2 hours. Subsequent treatments in the chamber are given at intervals of about 8 hours for the first 24 hours and then at intervals of 12 hours[38].

Outcome

The mortality rate from gas gangrene infection is approximately 25%. Some of the classical findings (haemolysis, renal failure and hypotension) occur late in the course of the illness and their presence may indicate a worse prognosis.

Anthrax
Aetiology

Worldwide there are about 100 000 cases of anthrax, mainly cutaneous, each year but very few if any occur in the UK or the rest of Europe. The disease is caused by a Gram-positive rod, *Bacillus anthracis*, which can form spores that survive for many years and can contaminate hides, hooves, hair and bones of cattle and goats. Live bacilli are found in the tissue of infected animals. Transmission to humans occurs in a variety of ways: skin contact with hides or meat, inhalation of spores or ingestion of infected meat, causing skin, respiratory or gastrointestinal disease, respectively, and finally laboratory-acquired infection. Onset of symptoms occurs within 5 days. Despite its rarity, anthrax remains of some importance for ICU staff because of the life-threatening nature of the condition and its relevance in the context of biological warfare.

Presentation

Cutaneous anthrax is relatively benign and presents as a red macule or papule at the site of contact. This develops into a pruritic vesicle, satellite lesions appear and this is followed by ulceration and a black eschar. Occasionally the local lesion is severe and accompanied by general toxaemia.

Inhalational anthrax initially presents with a dry cough followed by improvement and then sudden onset of severe respiratory distress. The patient becomes very ill with cough, cyanosis, tachypnoea, fever, tachycardia and vomiting. There is massive swelling of the neck and chest wall, enlargement of the spleen and, if untreated, the patient can die within 24 hours.

Gastrointestinal anthrax presents as severe gastroenteritis with haemorrhage. Lesions may be present anywhere in the gut including the pharynx. Haematogenous spread can sometimes cause meningitis. The mortality rate is high.

Diagnosis

The cutaneous form may be diagnosed from the occupational history and clinically. Inhalational anthrax, which might present to an ICU but without a history of possible exposure, might go undiagnosed as severe pneumonia. The organisms can be identified from skin lesions which should be biopsied in cutaneous disease and may be cultured from blood in more systemic forms.

Management

The cutaneous form may resolve without treatment but benzylpenicillin is very effective; $2 \, \text{g day}^{-1}$ in divided doses should be given for mild cutaneous disease and $4-6 \, \text{g day}^{-1}$ for more severe infection. Chloramphenicol can be used in cases of penicillin allergy[39]. Severe systemic disease will require organ support and maintenance of oxygen delivery. Prevention is by elimination of the disease from animals but immunization is available for those who have occupational exposure.

Key points

- Multiple trauma represents an important and frequent indication for admission to the ICU and a multidisciplinary approach is recommended to ensure optimal care.
- In trauma and burns, prompt resuscitation and surgical management (e.g. removal of devitalized tissue) reduce the risk of infection.
- Appropriate vaccines and long-term prophylactic antibiotics are indicated for all patients following splenectomy.
- In necrotizing fasciitis, rapidly progressive severe necrosis of subcutaneous tissues is accompanied by toxaemia commonly caused by group A streptococci (*Streptococcus pyogenes*).
- Necrosis of muscle due to toxigenic clostridial infection is the characteristic feature of gas gangrene.

REFERENCES

1. Vincent J-L, Bihari D, Suter P et al. (1995) The prevalence of nosocomial infection in intensive care units in Europe. Results of the European Prevalence of Infection in Intensive Care (EPIC) Study. EPIC International Advisory Committee. *Journal of the American Medical Association* **274**: 639–644.
2. Rotondo MF, Zonies DH (1997) The damage control sequence and underlying logic. *Surgical Clinics of North America* **77**: 761–777.
3. Barquist E, Kirton OC, Civetta JM (1998) Gastric intramucosal pH in the assessment of adequacy of resuscitation after trauma. *Current Opinion in Critical Care* **4**: 259–262.
4. Barquist E, Kirton OC, Windsor J et al. (1998) The impact of antioxidant and splanchnic-directed therapy on persistent uncorrected gastric mucosal pH in the critically ill trauma patient. *Journal of Trauma* **44**: 355–360.
5. Nielson VG, Tan S, Baird M et al. (1996) Gastric intramucosal pH and multiple organ injury: impact of ischaemia–reperfusion and xanthine oxidase. *Critical Care Medicine* **24**: 1339–1344.
6. Kirton OC, Windsor J, Wedderburn R et al. (1998) Failure of splanchnic resuscitation in the acutely injured trauma patient correlates with multiple system organ failure and length of stay in the ICU. *Chest* **113**: 1064–1069.

7. Offner PJ, Moore EE, Burt JM et al. (1998) Staged laparotomy for the lethal syndrome of postinjury hypothermia, acidosis and coagulopathy. *Current Opinion in Critical Care* **4**: 245–250.
8. Gustilo RB, Merkow RL, Templeman D (1990) The management of open fractures. *Journal of Bone and Joint Surgery* **72A**: 299–304.
9. Bumaschny E (1998) The abdominal compartment syndrome. *Current Opinion in Critical Care* **4**: 236–244.
10. Martin RR, Byrne M (1998) Postoperative care and complications of damage control surgery. *Surgical Clinics of North America* **77**: 929–942.
11. Low DE, McGeer A (1998) Skin and soft tissue infection; necrotising fasciitis. *Current Opinion in Infectious Diseases* **11**: 119–123.
12. Talan DA, Citron DM, Abrahamian FM et al. (1999) Bacteriological analysis of infected dog and cat bites. *New England Journal of Medicine* **340**: 85–92.
13. Department of Health, Welsh Office, Scottish Office, Department of Health and the Department of Health and Social Services (Northern Ireland) (1996) *Immunisation Against Infectious Diseases*. HMSO, London.
14. Lew DP, Waldvogel FA (1997) Osteomyelitis. *New England Journal of Medicine* **336**: 999–1007.
15. Dua HS (1998) Bacterial keratitis in the critically ill and comatose patient. *Lancet* **351**: 387–388.
16. Hassan IJ, MacGowan AP, Cook SD (1992) Endophthalmitis at the Bristol Eye Hospital; an 11 year review of 47 patients. *Journal of Hospital Infection* **22**: 271–278.
17. Andrews V (1995) Antibiotic treatment of ophthalmic infection: new developments. *Journal of Hospital Infection* **30** (Suppl): 268–274.
18. Timms J, Humphreys H (1997) Antibiotic prophylaxis in the intensive care unit. *Current Anaesthesia and Critical Care* **8**: 133–138.
19. Infection in Neurosurgery Working Party of the British Society of Antimicrobial Chemotherapy (1994) Antimicrobial prophylaxis in neurosurgery and after head injury. *Lancet* **344**: 1547–1551.
20. Malangoni MA, Jacobs TG (1992) Antibiotic prophylaxis for injured patients. *Infectious Disease Clinics of North America* **6**: 627–642.
21. Stoutenbeek CP, van Saene HKF, Miranda DR et al. (1984) The effect of selective decontamination of the digestive tract on colonisation and infection rate in multiple trauma patients. *Intensive Care Medicine* **10**: 185–192.
22. Ledingham IMcA, Alcock SR, Eastaway AT et al. (1988) Triple regimen of selective decontamination of the digestive tract, systemic cefotaxime, and microbiological surveillance for prevention of acquired infection in intensive care. *Lancet* **i**: 785–790.
23. Quinto B, Albanese J, Bues-Charbit M et al. (1996) Selective decontamination of the digestive tract in multiple trauma patients. A prospective, double-blind, randomized, placebo controlled study. *Chest* **109**: 765–772.
24. D'Amico R, Pifferi S, Leonetti C et al. (1998) Effectiveness of antibiotic prophylaxis in critically ill adult patients: systematic review of randomised controlled trials. *British Medical Journal* **316**: 1275–1285.
25. Working Party of the British Committee for Standards in Haematology Clinical Haematology Task Force (1996) Guidelines for the prevention and treatment of infection in patients with an absent or dysfunctional spleen. *British Medical Journal* **312**: 430–434.
26. Monafo WW (1996) Initial management of burns. *New England Journal of Medicine* **335**: 1581–1586.

27. Smith DJ, Thomson PD, Garner WL *et al.* (1994) Burn wounds: infection and healing. *American Journal of Surgery* **167** (Suppl 1A): 46S–48S.

28. Deitch EA (1990) The management of burns. *New England Journal of Medicine* **323**: 1249–1253.

29. Mackie DP, van Hertum WAJ, Schumberg T *et al.* (1992) Prevention of infection in burns: preliminary experience with selective decontamination of the digestive tract in patients with extensive burns. *Journal of Trauma* **32**: 570.

30. Brook I, Frazier EH (1995) Clinical and microbiological features of necrotising fasciitis. *Journal of Clinical Microbiology* **33**: 2382–2387.

31. Kaul R, McGeer A, Low DE *et al.* (1997) Population-based surveillance for group A streptococcal necrotising fasciitis: clinical features, prognostic indicators and microbiologic analysis of 77 cases. *American Journal of Medicine* **103**: 18–24.

32. Davies HD, McGeer A, Schwarz B *et al.* (1996) Invasive group A streptococcal infections in Ontario, Canada. *New England Journal of Medicine* **335**: 547–554.

33. Holm SE (1996) Invasive group A streptococcal infections. *New England Journal of Medicine* **335**: 590–591.

34. Burge TS, Watson JD (1994) Necrotising fasciitis. Be bloody, bold and resolute. *British Medical Journal* **308**: 1453–1454.

35. Ringel AF, Jameson GL, Foster ES (1995) Diarrhoea in the intensive care patient. *Intensive Care Clinics* **11**: 465–477.

36. Pizzorno R, Bonini F, Doneli A *et al.* (1997) Hyperbaric oxygen therapy in the treatment of Fournier's disease in 11 male patients. *Journal of Urology* **158**: 837–840.

37. Norrby-Tegland A, Kaul R, Low DE *et al.* (1996) Evidence for the presence of streptococcal superantigen neutralizing antibodies in normal polyspecific IgG (IVIG). *Infection and Immunity* **64**: 5395–5398.

38. Sussman M, Boriello SP, Taylor DJ (1998) Gas gangrene and other clostridial infections. In: *Topley and Wilson's Microbiology and Microbial Infections, vol. 3, Bacterial Infections* (eds Collier L, Balows A, Sussman M), pp. 669–691. Arnold, London.

39. Quinn CP, Turnbull PCB (1998) Anthrax. In: *Topley and Wilson's Microbiology and Microbial Infections, vol. 3, Bacterial Infections* (eds Collier L, Balows A, Sussman M), pp. 799–818. Arnold, London.

11 Central nervous system infections

The annual incidence of bacterial meningitis in the UK is 3–4 cases per 100 000 population with more than 50% of cases occurring in children under 5 years of age[1]. In the USA, *Streptococcus pneumoniae* is now the commonest pathogen with an incidence of 1.1 per 100 000 and with a 21% mortality rate[2]. Patients with infection of the central nervous system (CNS) are almost always critically ill and require intensive care early in the clinical course. Meningitis and encephalitis are the two commonest and most important CNS infections although there may be a degree of overlap between the two, for example *Listeria* infection. Other infections are much less common but it is important to recognize and confirm diagnosis promptly so that specific treatment can be started as soon as possible.

MENINGITIS

Aetiology

The commonest causes of bacterial meningitis in adults are *Neisseria meningitidis* (meningococcus) and *S. pneumoniae* (pneumococcus). There has been a striking decrease in meningitis due to *Haemophilus influenzae* in children less than 4 years of age during recent years following the introduction of *H. influenzae* type b (Hib) vaccination, but this has been accompanied by a rise in the incidence of meningococcal disease[1]. Meningococcal meningitis has a peak incidence in the first 2 years of life and then decreases, but has a second peak in older teenagers and young adults which has increased in recent years due to an increase in serogroup C disease.

Viral meningitis (due to enteroviruses such as coxsackie, echovirus, poliovirus and mumps virus) is much more common than bacterial meningitis but the latter is more serious and more likely to warrant admission to the intensive care unit (ICU). Other organisms that occasionally cause meningitis include *Myobacterium tuberculosis*, Gram-negative bacteria, staphylococci, *Listeria monocytogenes* and *Leptospira* spp. In patients infected with human immunodeficiency virus (HIV), organisms such as *Cryptococcus neoformans* may infect the CNS (see Chapter 12). Nosocomial bacterial meningitis due to other Gram-negative bacilli and Gram-positive cocci is becoming more important. Ventriculostomy catheters used for cerebrospinal fluid (CSF) drainage or monitoring intracranial pressure can become a source of infection, with meningitis or ventriculitis occurring in up to 10% of cases particularly if the devices are left in for 5 days or more (see below).

Pathogenesis

An acute inflammatory process occurs in the meninges, which in severe cases also involves the brain and vasculature. Bacterial cell lysis results in release of endotoxin in meningococcal and *Haemophilus* infection with subsequent release of cytokines, e.g. interleukin 1 (IL-1), IL-6, tumour necrosis factor (TNF). Waage *et al.* found a correlation between TNF concentrations in serum and fatal outcome in patients with meningococcal disease[3]. Activation of polymorphonuclear leukocytes occurs with adhesion to endothelium and release of toxic oxygen radicals and nitric oxide which all impair the blood–brain barrier. Vasogenic oedema contributes to raised intracranial pressure[4]. In animals, cytokine release is increased by antibiotics that lyse cell walls and is reduced by prior administration of TNF antibody or dexamethasone. As yet, however, these findings have no diagnostic or therapeutic implications.

Presentation

Meningitis is usually associated with the signs of meningism, which are headache, neck stiffness, photophobia and fever. Signs of raised intracranial pressure (papilloedema, vomiting, drowsiness) are more common with bacterial meningitis and loss of consciousness may be very rapid. Unfortunately the prodromal features can be non-specific, making early diagnosis difficult, but a delay in diagnosis and treatment of bacterial meningitis increases the risk of death and permanent neurological damage. Meningococcal septicaemia has a classical presentation accompanied by a purpuric rash which occurs in approximately 70% of patients (Plate 11). The bacteraemia may be profound with disseminated intravascular coagulation (DIC) and septic shock leading to multi-organ failure. The circulatory collapse may be secondary to adrenal haemorrhage (the Waterhouse–Friederichsen syndrome).

Pneumococcal meningitis is commoner in the elderly and chronically debilitated. It is accompanied by a high incidence of early seizures and late neurological damage (hydrocephalus, deafness and epilepsy) and the mortality rate is high.

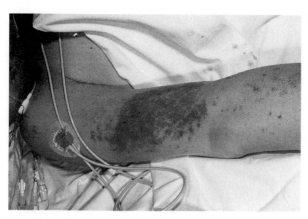

Plate 11 Purpuric rash.

Diagnosis

Diagnosis is usually confirmed by microbiological examination of CSF obtained by lumbar puncture, but this is inadvisable in the presence of signs of raised intracranial pressure or if the patient exhibits focal neurological signs.

Two sets of blood cultures and a throat swab (to detect carriage which is suggestive but not diagnostic) should always be taken from any patient presenting with a febrile illness where CNS infection is suspected. Appropriate specimens are listed in Table 11.1.

Additional investigations include the polymerase chain reaction (PCR) on specimens of CSF or blood to detect bacterial nucleic acid, aspirates of purpuric lesions for Gram stain and one or more serum samples for meningococcal antibodies, which will retrospectively confirm the diagnosis. These investigations not only help to confirm a diagnosis but also assist in the management of contacts. Meningococcal PCR is currently available in the UK at the Meningococcal Reference Unit and in other countries. Pneumococcal PCR is also being developed and may assist in detecting resistance genes[5].

The CSF findings in the various types of meningitis are summarized in Table 11.2 but there is some overlap between the various categories.

Table 11.1 Appropriate specimens for the investigation of suspected meningococcal disease.

1. CSF – microscopy and culture

2. Blood for culture should always be obtained even if parenteral penicillin has been given before hospital admission

3. Non-culture diagnosis. If CSF microscopy fails to identify *N. meningitidis* in a suspected case, part of the remaining specimen should be submitted for polymerase chain reaction (PCR) investigation with an EDTA blood specimen (2.5–5 ml) taken on admission and sent immediately. Heparinized blood specimens are unsuitable. If a delay of more than 24 hours in dispatching samples is anticipated, the blood or serum should be frozen in the laboratory. Paired serum specimens (at least 0.5 ml) for serology should be obtained for retrospective diagnosis of meningococcal disease: to detect IgM and IgG antibodies directed against meningococcal outer membrane proteins

4. Throat swabs (a sweep of the pharyngeal wall and tonsils) should be taken from all patients as a positive result is suggestive of the aetiology if blood and CSF are culture negative

5. If the patient has a haemorrhagic skin rash (petechiae, purpura or larger areas of haemorrhage), lesions can be lanced and a smear made for microscopy

Table 11.2   CSF findings in meningitis.

	Normal	Bacterial	Viral	Tuberculosis
Appearance	Clear	Purulent	Clear/ opalescent	Clear/ opalescent
Cell count	0–5 mm^{-3} (lymphocytes)	5–2000 mm^{-3} (neutrophils)	5–500 mm^{-3} (lymphocytes)	5–1000 mm^{-3} (lymphocytes)
Glucose	60% of blood level	Low, <60% of blood level	Normal	Low
Protein	0.1–0.4 g l^{-1}	>1.0 g l^{-1}	0.5–0.9 g l^{-1}	>1.0 g l^{-1}
Microscopy	—	Bacteria may be seen on Gram stain	—	Bacteria very occasionally seen on Ziehl–Neelsen stain

Management

Patients may present with profound septic shock and acidosis and may die within hours of arrival in hospital. They present a major challenge for the ICU, requiring immediate invasive monitoring, rapid fluid resuscitation, inotropic therapy and often empirical haemofiltration. Adrenal insufficiency may require corticosteroid replacement. The generalized vascular damage that can occur often requires later amputation of digits or limbs.

When bacterial meningitis is strongly suspected but microscopy is negative and the results of culture and other investigations are awaited, antibiotics must be started without delay because of the potentially severe consequences. Empirical treatment must include one or more antibiotics active against the most common causes and include agents that penetrate the blood–brain barrier. Cefotaxime (i.v., 2 g 4–6-hourly) will cover the most common causes pending culture and sensitivity results. Ampicillin (i.v., 2 g 4-hourly) should be added if *Listeria* is suspected (Table 11.3).

Meningococcal meningitis

Meningococcal meningitis is usually part of a septicaemic illness. It is the common form of bacterial meningitis in young adults. Optimal treatment is with high-dose benzylpenicillin (i.v., 2.4 g 4–6-hourly) in the absence of a history of anaphylaxis (or cefotaxime, 2 g 4–6-hourly, in those allergic to penicillin). Antimicrobial treatment should continue for 7 days. Close contacts of the patient should be treated in consultation with public health doctors or microbiologists

Table 11.3 Guidelines for antibiotic treatment of meningitis.

Infection	Suggested antibacterial intravenous therapy (adult dose)	Comment
	Initial blind therapy with cefotaxime, 2 g 4-hourly	
Meningococci	Benzylpenicillin, 2.4 g 4–6-hourly Cefotaxime, 2 g 4-hourly, if allergic to penicillin	Give rifampicin for 2 days (adult 600 mg b.i.d.) or ciprofloxacin, 500 mg once, before hospital discharge to reduce nasopharyngeal carriage
Pneumococci	Benzylpenicillin, 2.4 g 4–6-hourly Cefotaxime, 2 g 4-hourly, if allergic to penicillin	
Listeria	Ampicillin, 2 g 4-hourly, plus gentamicin, 5 mg kg^{-1} daily (serum levels of gentamicin require regular monitoring)	Measure creatinine level within 6 hours of first dose of gentamicin

with rifampicin (600 mg b.i.d. for 2 days) or a single dose of ciprofloxacin (500 mg) to eradicate nasal carriage of the organism. The index patient should also receive rifampicin or ciprofloxacin as neither benzylpenicillin nor cefotaxime is very effective in eradicating upper airway carriage. Health care workers involved in the care of the patient do not require prophylaxis unless engaged in mouth-to-mouth resuscitation or where intubation has been difficult resulting in heavy aerolization of the patient's secretions.

Pneumococcal meningitis

Benzylpenicillin (2.4 g 4-hourly) remains the treatment of choice for sensitive organisms but resistant strains are emerging in some parts of the world[6, 7] and a third-generation cephalosporin is now the recommended therapy in many countries pending confirmation of penicillin sensitivity. In the USA, up to 25% of invasive strains are resistant to penicillin (7% highly resistant) and 9% of isolates are resistant to cefotaxime. It is difficult to obtain adequate CSF concentrations of antibiotics against multiply antibiotic-resistant pneumococci; at present vancomycin, rifampicin or meropenem are most prescribed. Clinicians should be aware of local resistance patterns and therapy with a cephalosporin (cefotaxime or ceftriaxone) and vancomycin with dexamethasone is recommended[8]. Plasma levels of vancomycin greater than 30 mg l^{-1} should be achieved but those >60 mg l^{-1} avoided. A repeat lumbar puncture should be undertaken to review eradication and, in the event of failure, rifampicin should be substituted for vancomycin[9].

Listeria *meningitis*

This should be considered especially in pregnant women or in immuno-suppressed hosts such as patients with lymphoma. Cephalosporins have poor activity against *Listeria*. The antibiotic treatment of choice is ampicillin (i.v., 2 g 4–6-hourly; considered superior to penicillin) and gentamicin (i.v., 5 mg kg^{-1} day^{-1}), using serum levels to monitor for toxicity. Treatment should be continued for 21 days[10].

Nosocomial meningitis

Extended-spectrum cephalosporins are active against most Gram-negative bacilli but sensitivity must be obtained in every case. Ceftazidime should be used for immunocompromised patients who may have *P. aeruginosa*. A systemically administered aminoglycoside may be added. Sensitive staphylococci may be treated with flucloxacillin but often the only reliable treatment for methicillin-resistant *Staphylococcus aureus* (MRSA) is vancomycin[6]. Intrathecal adminis-tration is indicated where a strain of MRSA is present. Where the isolate is susceptible, chloramphenicol may be considered as an alternative. Enterococci require a combination of a cell wall-active antibiotic and an aminoglycoside; in difficult cases the latter can be given intrathecally.

Antibiotic therapy for bacterial meningitis should continue for a minimum of 7 days unless otherwise specified but should continue for 10 days for *Haemophilus* meningitis and uncomplicated pneumococcal meningitis. How-ever, changes in the aetiology of meningitis, the spread of penicillin-resistant pneumococci and the possible emergence of antibiotic-resistant meningococci require careful surveillance[2, 6, 11], but at present high-dose cefotaxime (i.v., 2 mg 4–6 hourly) or ceftriaxone (iv., up to 4 mg daily) remain the drugs of choice for empirical therapy.

Corticosteroids

A recent meta-analysis still supports the use of dexamethasone in children with *H. influenzae* meningitis, which if given early in the illness reduces hearing loss[12]. Trials in children with bacterial meningitis showed that compared to placebo dexamethasone adjuvant treatment resulted in a shorter febrile period and reduced the incidence of deafness and other neurological complications 1 year later. Most of the evidence for benefit from steroid therapy relates to *H. influenzae* and *S. pneumoniae* infection but, as the pathophysiology of neuronal damage is similar for all types of meningitis, current recommendations are to treat all cases of suspected bacterial meningitis with dexamethasone (0.2 mg kg^{-1} three times daily)[8, 13]. This treatment is not recommended for meningococcal septicaemia although in septic shock there may be impaired adrenocortical function and many intensivists would give 100 mg hydrocortisone followed by an infusion of 10 mg hour^{-1}.

Public health

Even before laboratory confirmation, cases of meningitis must be notified to public health or other appropriate authorities on clinical diagnosis to facilitate the implementation of chemoprophylaxis and to detect clusters or small outbreaks. Cases of meningitis are a cause of major concern among members of the public, who may direct enquiries to ICU staff, who in turn should usually pass these on to public health doctors or medical microbiologists. Confirmation of the aetiology by the laboratory may assist further preventive measures such as use of meningococcal vaccine.

Adjunctive therapy

The raised intracranial pressure (ICP) and epileptiform convulsions which may occur in any form of meningitis require urgent treatment. Raised ICP should be treated by 10–15° head-up tilt (except in hypotensive patients), avoidance of constriction of the neck veins and optimal oxygenation. Cerebral perfusion pressure should be maintained at a minimum of 70 mmHg by ensuring normovolaemia or slight hypervolaemia and then adding inotropic drugs as necessary. Cerebral ischaemia must be avoided and it is preferable to avoid hyperventilation, which temporarily reduces cerebral blood flow, as a mechanism for reducing ICP. The osmotic diuretic mannitol reduces brain water and in this respect may occasionally be useful treatment provided consequent electrolyte abnormalities are corrected. It should be given in an initial dose of $0.5\,g\,kg^{-1}$ and thereafter at $0.25\,g\,kg^{-1}$. Convulsions are usually treated acutely with diazepam or midazolam (i.v., up to 20 mg) and then with phenytoin (i.v., using a loading dose of $17\,mg\,kg^{-1}$ given slowly, then 300–400 mg daily). The likelihood of drug interactions is high owing to its metabolism via cytochrome P450, so drug concentration monitoring is recommended. The management of bacterial meningitis in adults has recently been comprehensively reviewed[14].

Outcome

Outcome depends upon early diagnosis and management[15, 16]. Prognosis for patients with bacterial meningitis who require intensive care is very poor, with less than 50% survival in a recently published series[13].

CEREBROSPINAL SHUNT INFECTIONS

Infection is one of the most serious complications of CSF shunt surgery, often required for the management of hydrocephalus. Rates of infection have improved in recent years and are now between 5 and 10% in most centres[17]. Shunt infection may involve infection of the wound (incision), the meninges (meningitis), peritoneum after a ventriculoperitoneal shunt or the actual shunt apparatus.

Aetiology and pathogenesis

Bacteria commonly present on the skin such as staphylococci and coryneforms are the most common cause of infection and are often introduced at the time of surgery. Internal shunt infections, where pathogens colonize the lumen of the shunt, are more common than external shunt infections. External infections may, however, be polymicrobial and are usually caused by *S. aureus* and aerobic Gram-negative bacilli[17]. Following surgery, the implanted shunt is almost immediately coated with a film or slime composed of serum and extracellular polysaccharides originating from bacteria. The resulting biofilm facilitates the persistence of infection and renders the penetration of antibiotics difficult. Risk factors that increase the risk of infection include younger patients (perhaps indicating an immature immune system), poor condition of the skin and concurrent infections elsewhere[17].

Presentation
Fever, chills, irritability, neck stiffness, headache and vomiting in a patient with a CSF shunt should prompt the diagnosis. Infection with *S. aureus* or cerebritis is often more acute in its presentation and may be accompanied by bacteraemia. There may be local evidence of wound infection and abdominal tenderness may suggest peritonitis.

Diagnosis
Microbiological examination of the CSF obtained through the shunt or directly from the ventricles is the key to making the diagnosis, and often repeated samples are required to confirm the aetiology (*Staphylococcus epidermidis* can occasionally contaminate CSF and other specimens) and to monitor the response to antibiotic therapy. The peripheral white cell count may be raised and computed tomography (CT) or magnetic resonance imaging (MRI) may indicate enlarged ventricles due to obstruction, requiring the insertion of an external ventricular drain (EVD). Research is ongoing to develop a reliable serological assay that can assist in diagnosis and help to avoid the unnecessary removal of shunts. However, when removed, the shunt should be carefully transported to the laboratory and cultured to guide the choice and method of administration of antibiotics.

Management
Close cooperation between neurosurgeons, ICU staff and medical microbiologists is essential to optimize therapy. CSF shunt removal with antibiotics administered via an EVD carries the highest cure rate and the lowest mortality rate[17]. The EVD which often remains *in situ* for a week or longer facilitates drainage and control of intracranial pressure, allows the taking of daily CSF specimens to monitor response to treatment and provides the opportunity to administer antibiotics directly into the ventricles. These benefits outweigh the risk of secondary infection of the EVD and the current consensus is that immediate or early replacement of the shunt may be associated with relapse of infection. The choice of antibiotics is largely influenced by the sensitivity of the pathogen recovered (many isolates of *S. epidermidis* are multiply antibiotic resistant) and penetration of the agent into the CSF. For suspected Gram-positive infection, e.g. *S. epidermidis* and coryneforms, intraventricular vancomycin (20 mg daily;

a lower dose should be given if the CSF volume is reduced) should be administered through the clamped EVD with rifampicin (i.v. or oral, 600 mg twice daily) to be continued until the patient is reshunted[18]. Intravenous flucloxacillin should be added if infection with *S. aureus* is confirmed and the isolate is sensitive. Both aminoglycosides and cephalosporins are indicated for infection due to aerobic Gram-negative infection and the former may need to be administered intrathecally. Reshunting may be possible at 7–10 days but treatment is usually recommended for 10–14 days.

Prevention

Prevention of infection is based upon good surgical practice at the time of shunt insertion, antimicrobial chemoprophylaxis and the development of shunt materials that are less prone to infection (e.g. the incorporation of antibacterial compounds). Prophylactic antibiotics are often administered despite little scientific evidence in their favour. Advice from the Working Party of the British Society of Antimicrobial Chemotherapy should be followed for antimicrobial prophylaxis in neurosurgery and after head injury[19]. A second-generation cephalosporin such as cefuroxime is recommended for clean non-implant procedures and co-amoxiclav for clean-contaminated procedures. There is no definitive recommendation for CSF shunt procedures but vancomycin and gentamicin instilled into the ventricles during surgery are used by some surgeons in complicated patients with the aim of reducing infection.

ENCEPHALITIS

Patients with severe meningitis may have secondary encephalitis but most commonly encephalitis is a primary disease, usually viral, involving the cerebral cortex, often with an acute alteration in mental state and convulsions. Encephalitis is clinically less clear cut than meningitis and some or all of the symptoms of meningitis (e.g. headache) with loss of consciousness or changes in mentation may suggest the diagnosis. In recent years the incidence has fallen with the elimination worldwide of smallpox and the introduction of immunization against measles, mumps and rubella[20, 21].

Aetiology

Herpes simplex is a common cause of acute encephalitis (HSE). The virus, usually herpes simplex type 1, preferentially attacks the frontal and temporal lobes and is believed to result from reactivation of virus latent in the cranial nerve ganglia. The annual incidence is between 1 in 250 000 to 1 per million population. Other viral causes of encephalitis include varicella-zoster, measles, mumps, cytomegalovirus, Epstein–Barr virus, arbovirus and rabies. Arthropod-borne arboviruses should be considered in patients who have recently come from areas where these infections are prevalent (e.g. California and St Louis encephalitis). Post-infectious encephalomyelitis caused by measles, rubella and varicella may closely resemble acute encephalitis and MRI scans may help to differentiate. Tuberculosis, syphilis, toxoplasmosis and Lyme disease may all be associated with encephalitis but this is not the most common presentation of these infections.

Presentation

Acute deterioration of consciousness level occurs with fever and convulsions and sometimes focal signs, which suggest the diagnosis[22]. There may be a history of a prodromal illness with flu-like symptoms. Evidence of current or recent orolabial or genital herpes has no diagnostic implications. Ninety per cent of patients with HSE have signs suggestive of a localized lesion in one or both temporal lobes[22].

Diagnosis

Unlike most causes of viral encephalitis, HSE does respond to antiviral drugs, so diagnosis is crucial. Abnormalities in the frontal and temporal areas may be detected on electroencephalography (EEG) or CT. Serial investigations should be used to follow the course of the disease. Previously the diagnosis was confirmed by brain biopsy and differential serum/CSF antibody levels, but increasingly PCR for herpes simplex virus type 1 and type 2 nucleic acid in CSF is available[23, 24]. Even if antiviral therapy has already commenced on suspicion of the diagnosis, HSE can still be detected for up to 5 days thereafter. With the use of PCR, it is becoming apparent that herpes simplex virus type 2 is more common as a cause than was previously thought[24].

Varicella-zoster virus encephalitis has become more common with the increase in AIDS. Vascular damage occurs mainly in large vessels with secondary infection of glial cells. The differential diagnosis of viral encephalitis includes:

1. Vasculitis
2. Sarcoidosis
3. Alcoholic encephalopathy
4. Metabolic encephalopathy
5. Toxins
6. Reye's syndrome
7. Brain abscess
8. Brain tumour
9. Intracranial haemorrhage
10. Tuberculous and fungal meningitis

Investigations should therefore include liver function tests, blood cultures, plasma samples for antibody levels, a toxin screen and venereal disease reference laboratory (VDRL) screen for syphilis, although this is increasingly uncommon as a cause. However, a CT scan will often have excluded some of these, including intracranial masses such as haemorrhage and neoplasia. Lumbar puncture should be considered if intracranial pressure is not raised. CSF specimens should be sent for cytology, routine microbiology, tuberculosis and fungal cultures and for PCR to detect viruses[24]. Typically CSF protein is raised and there is a lymphocytosis but the glucose concentration is normal and both Gram stain and culture are negative.

Management

As soon as the diagnosis of herpes encephalitis is suspected, treatment with aciclovir (i.v., 10 mg kg^{-1} 8-hourly) should be commenced and continued for 14 days or until another diagnosis is made[25]. Aciclovir is of most benefit if started before brain necrosis is well established and a recent algorithm for diagnosis and treatment of suspected HSE is provided by a European Union consensus group[26]. Aciclovir may be replaced shortly by famciclovir which has enhanced bioavailability. At present, however, there are no reports of resistance to aciclovir and it also has some activity against both varicella-zoster and Epstein–Barr encephalitis.

Ganciclovir is the treatment of choice for cytomegalovirus (CMV) encephalitis and amantidine administered very early in the course of the illness may be of some benefit in patients with encephalitis due to influenza A. Excessive dehydration should be avoided to reduce renal toxicity from aciclovir and the dose should be modified in renal failure. Intensive care and supportive therapy only minimally increases survival in rabies virus infection. Neither antiviral therapy nor immunoglobulin have improved outcome.

CEREBRAL ABSCESS

Aetiology

Brain abscess is a well-known complication of brain trauma, dental and nasal infections, chronic suppurative otitis media, cyanotic congenital heart disease and occasionally meningitis. The anatomical location is often determined by predisposing factors which in turn influence aetiology. For example, sinusitis predisposes to frontal lobe abscesses caused by streptococci and anaerobes. Abscesses that complicate infective endocarditis are often multiple and are most commonly caused by *S. aureus*. Organ transplantation is now a fairly standard procedure but, with the advent of more sophisticated agents to prevent organ rejection, the threat of opportunistic infection including brain abscess becomes greater and must be considered in the diagnosis and management. A review by Hagensee *et al.* of brain abscesses after bone marrow transplantation showed that fungi were isolated in 92% of cases and the mortality rate was 97%[27]. Furthermore, there was no clinical improvement with antifungal therapy.

Incidence

Two to four bacterial brain abscesses occur per million population each year with a peak incidence in children aged 4–7 years and in adults during the third decade[28].

Presentation and pathogenesis

The features are those of any expanding lesion in the brain which include headache, drowsiness, vomiting and, less frequently, localizing signs and fitting. The patient may be febrile with a raised white cell count. This is not a very common condition, hence it may be missed in hospitals that are not referral centres and that consequently may not see cases very frequently. Undiagnosed, the patient deteriorates with a decreasing Glasgow Coma Score. Clinical features vary with the site and size of the lesion, the infecting organism and the host response, but the illness is usually subacute and evolves over days or weeks. In about 50% of patients there is a single lesion, and overall the most common sites of infection are in the frontal and parietal regions. Approximately 25% of patients with cerebral abscesses have no documented antecedent infections. The average overall incidence of neurological complications including brain abscess in patients with infective endocarditis is 30%, with the vast majority of these occurring in patients with left heart valvular disease. The incidence of embolic events tends to be higher in cases of endocarditis caused by more virulent organisms such as *S. aureus* and the Enterobacteriaceae.

Diagnosis

CSF examination is insufficient for establishing the diagnosis. Significant advances have been made recently in the diagnosis and management of both brain abscesses and subdural empyema following the availability of CT and MRI scanning, resulting in a decrease in mortality (Figures 11.1 and 11.2). These greatly facilitate early recognition and treatment by aspiration of pus through a burr hole. Immediate Gram staining followed by culture of pus to establish sensitivity of the organisms will guide therapy and local antibiotics can be instilled. The most common bacteria associated with brain abscess are streptococci (aerobic, α- and β-haemolytic), *S. aureus*, *S. pneumoniae*, *Proteus vulgaris*, enterococci and increasingly *Bacteroides* spp. and anaerobic streptococci.

Management
Specific

Treatment consists of surgery to drain pus, and administration of intravenous antibiotics. Surgery is usually performed on abscesses larger than 2.5 cm or on those situated in critical areas of the brain or causing significant mass effects. Any abscess that enlarges after 2 weeks of antibiotics or that fails to shrink after 3–4 weeks of antibiotics should again be aspirated or excised[28]. Craniotomy with primary extirpation and resection of the abscess membrane, burr-hole craniotomy with puncture or insertion of a drain, marsupialization or stereotactic aspiration, are all possible therapeutic approaches. Stereotactic surgery using an endoscope to aspirate the abscess contents leaving the abscess membrane *in situ* is a recent technique.

Antibiotic therapy is governed by microbial diagnosis, antimicrobial pharmacokinetics and antibiotic susceptibility patterns to ensure sterilization of brain tissue. Antibiotics may be administered intravenously for up to 6–8 weeks but the duration will depend upon the causative organism and the initial response to treatment. Empirical antibiotic treatment should be started pending the results of culture and sensitivity. Treatment should include those antibiotics that cross the blood–brain barrier and are likely to be active against the commonest

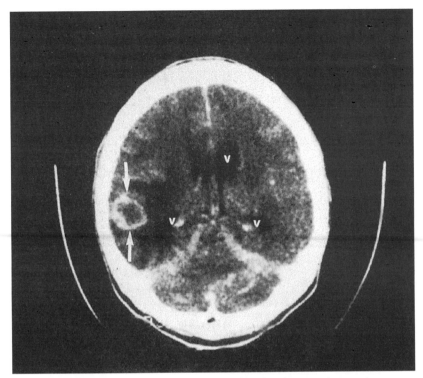

Figure 11.1. Contrast-enhanced CT scan of brain abscess (arrows).

pathogens. An initial antibiotic regimen might include cefotaxime (i.v., 2 g 4-hourly) with metronidazole (i.v., 500 mg 8-hourly). An alternative in those patients with a genuine history of penicillin allergy is chloramphenicol, despite the potential adverse effects on bone marrow function, as this agent penetrates very well into the CNS. The aminoglycosides have only a limited role, unless administered intrathecally, because of poor penetration of the brain. This combined approach involving surgery and antibiotics achieves cure rates of more than 90%, even in patients with multiple brain abscesses[29]. Bi-weekly CT or MRI is necessary to monitor patients closely for evidence of abscess enlargement, or failure to resolve despite antibiotics, prompting a further operation.

Supportive
Intensive care involves maintaining CNS homeostasis by control of intracranial pressure, maintenance of cerebral perfusion pressure and provision of systemic support.

Outcome
Successful clinical outcomes are not achieved in all patients who undergo image-guided stereotactic surgery as the initial procedure in the management of brain abscess. Factors associated with initial treatment failure include

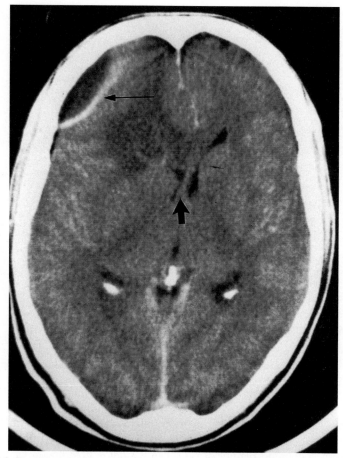

Figure 11.2 CT scan of subdural empyema (thin arrow) with space-occupying effects (thick arrow).

inadequate aspiration, lack of catheter drainage of larger abscesses, chronic immunosuppression, and inadequate antibiotic therapy. The overall mortality rate is about 10% but prognosis is largely determined by the clinical state at the time of presentation. Persistent convulsions occur in up to 50% of survivors. Recent studies suggest the most significant predictors of poor outcome are the patient's level of consciousness at presentation and the rapidity of disease progression prior to the initiation of treatment[28].

BOTULISM

Aetiology and pathogenesis
The main form of human botulism throughout the world is food-borne intoxication. Food-borne enterotoxin-mediated disease caused by *Clostridium botulinum* (botulism) is still common in the developing world, and is most

frequent in rural areas[30] as the heat-resistant spores survive food preservation. Wound botulism (after trauma or intravenous drug abuse) is rare and most of the documented cases have been described in the USA. In Europe, botulism remains a rare but serious disease that can be prevented by adequate preparation of food products[31]. A recent outbreak due to contaminated imported vegetable soup showed the importance of correct handling in industrial preservation processes and implementation of control mechanisms by rapid alert systems between countries[32].

Human botulism is normally limited to toxin types A, B and E, while types C and D predominate in avian and non-human mammalian species. All toxins are polypeptides of about 150 kDa that have similar structure and pharmacological action. The toxins act primarily at peripheral cholinergic synapses by blocking the invoked release of the neurotransmitter acetylcholine. Botulism outbreaks are a public health emergency requiring rapid recognition to prevent additional cases becoming infected, and in the individual patient to provide ventilation and early administration of antitoxin. Aerosolized *C. botulinum* toxin may be absorbed by the lungs and this could conceivably occur during a terrorist attack or during biological warfare.

Presentation

The neurotoxins produced by *C. botulinum* are the most potent neurotoxins known and are the causative agents of the neuroparalytic disease. The initial illness may be an afebrile one developing within 12–36 hours of eating contaminated food, usually tins of meat. Most patients, however, have only malaise and postural hypotension. About 3 days later, diplopia, bulbar signs and peripheral muscle weakness occur. The toxins act primarily at peripheral cholinergic synapses by irreversibly blocking the evoked release of acetylcholine. Patients may also present with cranial nerve palsies, descending paralysis and sometimes rapid onset of respiratory arrest. Infant botulism is characterized by a progressive symmetrical descending paralysis of cranial nerves with eventual involvement of axial and trunk muscle innervation, resulting in respiratory failure.

Diagnosis

The diagnosis of botulism is made clinically on the basis of the neurological signs and symptoms but may be missed if not considered in the differential diagnosis of patients with acute onset of paralysis. It is most often mistaken for Guillain–Barré syndrome but other toxins such as organophosphates should also be excluded. There may be a history of ingestion of contaminated food but this should not be relied upon. Diagnosis may be confirmed by tests that identify the toxin in the food source, the patient's blood or occasionally in faeces or vomitus, but diagnostic facilities are limited to national or international referral centres and any request must specify the suspected diagnosis. The application of PCR may improve detection but at present remains experimental.

Management

Treatment includes supportive intensive care[33] and the use of therapeutic antitoxin. Gastric lavage should be performed if contaminated food ingestion was recent and enemas can also be used to empty the lower gut. The use of magnesium should be avoided because of the additive effects with toxin. In wound botulism, surgical debridement reduces the toxin load. Ventilatory support is required for 2–8 weeks and in one case 7 months' ventilation was necessary before the return of ventilatory function[30]. The only specific treatment available is administration of antitoxin but this has no effect after the toxin has become bound to neural receptors. A single dose of equine antitoxin is administered depending on the toxin type[30]. Human antitoxin is becoming available but at present only for the treatment of infants. Intravenous benzylpenicillin will kill any remaining organisms in the gut.

Outcome

Death occurs in 5–10% of food-borne cases and in 15% of cases of wound botulism[30].

TETANUS

Aetiology

In Europe only carelessness in not maintaining acquired immunity (except perhaps in the elderly with reduced immunity) is responsible for the occurrence of tetanus. Between 1984 and 1995, 145 cases were documented in England and Wales, 53% in patients over 65 years of age. In the USA, 124 cases were reported during 1995–1997, only 13% of whom had received a course of tetanus toxoid[34, 35]. Adults over 60 years of age are most at risk and immunity is lowest amongst the elderly[34].

Pathogenesis

The illness is due to the action of an exotoxin (tetanospasmin) produced from spore-forming *Clostridium tetani*. *C. tetani* toxins are not absorbed from the bowel and are destroyed by digestive activity within the gut. Sites of entry are often minor wounds or varicose ulcers, although spores may gain entry through sites of arterial gangrene (diabetics), or after bowel and pelvic surgery, but in 10% or more of patients the entry site cannot be detected. Spores may very occasionally remain inactive within healed wounds and reactivate years later. It is exceptional for tetanus to occur in a subject who has had a booster tetanus toxoid injection within the last 10 years. From the site of infection the toxin spreads locally via the bloodstream and is absorbed at peripheral motor and autonomic nerve endings. The toxin spreads by intra-axonal retrograde transport, accumulates in the ventral root of the spinal cord and spreads to sensory and motor neurones. The severity of infection is affected by the quantity of toxin produced and the length of the neuronal pathway. No symptoms occur until the toxin has crossed the synaptic cleft to the presynaptic terminals of inhibitory spinal cord neurones. There it interferes with the release of inhibitory transmitters, causing synaptic disinhibition and producing pathological excitement at other neurones with simultaneous tetanospasms. The effects of toxin on the autonomic system are predominantly adrenergic stimulation.

Presentation

Muscle rigidity occurs resulting in trismus, risus sardonicus and dysphagia. Muscle spasms occur on mild stimulation. Lockjaw is not diagnostic of tetanus and local causes such as dental abscess, temporomandibular arthritis, neuroleptic drugs and hysteria should always be excluded. Muscle spasms spread to involve the trunk with opisthotonos, and fractures may occur during spasms[36]. Dysphagia and salivary drooling occur and glottic spasm may produce respiratory arrest. Profuse sweating, paroxysmal tachycardia, hypertension, hyperpyrexia and increased bronchial tone are features of autonomic disturbance.

Cephalic tetanus follows infected injuries of the head and neck, has a short incubation period and may present with cranial nerve palsies occurring in the absence of generalized tetanus.

Diagnosis

The diagnosis is largely clinical as the presence or absence of *C. tetani* in a wound neither confirms nor refutes the diagnosis. Furthermore, at the time of presentation the wound may have fully healed or not be noticed. The differential diagnoses includes hypocalcaemia, tetany, epilepsy, chorea and occasionally meningitis. Encephalitis should be excluded as this may also give rise to dystonia and abnormal movements.

Management
Eradication of infection

The wound should be fully debrided to reduce the bacterial and toxin load and benzylpenicillin (1.8–3.6 g day^{-1}) should be given in divided doses for more than 10 days. It has been suggested that metronidazole (i.v., 500 mg 6-hourly) may be preferred because of its comparable antimicrobial activity with reduced inhibitory transmitter antagonism[36].

Other measures require reference to the British National Formulary (BNF) or local equivalent but are summarized below.

Neutralization of free toxin

Before toxin is fixed to neuronal tissue, 150 IU kg^{-1} of hyperimmune human antitetanus immunoglobulin should be administered as a single dose but at multiple sites. This is less useful after the symptoms are well developed indicating that the toxin has not yet reached the spinal cord neurones. Tetanus immunoglobulin of human origin (HTIG) should be used selectively in addition to wound toilet, vaccine (which protects against subsequent disease) and benzyl-penicillin (or another appropriate antibiotic) for seriously contaminated wounds as prophylaxis. The dose of HTIG is 250 units increased to 500 units if more than 24 hours have elapsed or contamination is heavy. There is an intravenous preparation for use on a named-patient basis. HTIG is rarely required for patients with established immunity in whom protection may be achieved by a booster dose of vaccine if necessary (if the last booster was 10 or more years ago). Therefore HTIG should be considered only for patients not known to have received active immunization, whose wound was sustained more than 6 hours before treatment was started, or in those patients with puncture or heavily contaminated wounds with devitalized tissue. A precise evidence-based protocol remains to be established, but there is no special antitoxin available and most are contraindicated by the intrathecal route. A dose of adsorbed tetanus vaccine should be given at the same time as the tetanus immunoglobulin and the course of vaccine subsequently completed[20].

Intensive therapy
All oral feeding must be discontinued as further spasms may be provoked with the danger of aspiration of pharyngeal contents. Patients managed in the ICU will be intubated and ventilated with a nasogastric tube in situ through which enteral feeding is given. Owing to the protracted nature of the illness, tracheostomy is likely to be needed.

Outcome
Complications include high fever, continuous spasms, autonomic features, oliguria and death within 24–48 hours. Cardiac arrest may be precipitated by long periods of apnoea but death is late and secondary to pulmonary embolus in most cases. Recovery is slow and early muscle exercise is required to avoid stiffness of the joints and muscles; 3% of patients develop ossification around the joints. Nosocomial infection such as pneumonia may occur as with all patients who require prolonged intensive care. The mortality rate from mild tetanus is 10% but severe tetanus with generalized spasms has a rate approaching 50%, especially in countries where intensive care facilities are limited. In Europe the mortality rate from severe tetanus requiring intensive care is greater than 20%[37].

Prophylaxis
Complete vaccination against tetanus entails at least two injections of toxoid and a booster dose, which should be repeated at least every 10 years[20]. A further booster is required for wounds incurred more than 10 years after a course of tetanus toxoid. Therefore all patients presenting to their family doctor, the accident and emergency department or to the ICU should have their immunization status reviewed as tetanus is an easily preventable disease. Active immunization is also required during convalescence from acute disease as infection with tetanus does not necessarily confer protective immunity.

MISCELLANEOUS INFECTIONS

Transmissible spongiform encephalopathies

These diseases, which include kuru and Creutzfeldt–Jakob disease (CJD), are caused by infectious agents but usually present sporadically, although some are partly genetically determined. Basic molecular research combined with impressive population studies have recently confirmed that many of these infections are caused by novel infectious agents such as self-replicating proteins or prions which are very resistant to conventional methods of sterilization and treatments that inactivate nucleic acids and viruses[38].

In the UK, variant Creutzfeldt–Jakob disease (vCJD) was first diagnosed in 1995 and is currently believed to be linked to the outbreaks of bovine spongiform encephalopathy, which probably arose from the practice of feeding cows and calves meat and bone meal. This new variant is characterized by earlier age of onset, cerebellar signs, changes in behaviour rather than mentation and a longer interval from presentation to death[38, 39]. Until recently, diagnosis was often only confirmed at autopsy but the development of assays to detect specific protein markers in the CSF and tonsils[40] and improved imaging techniques are changing this. Histological examination of the brain and immunostaining for the protease-resistant protein associated with the disease are the gold standards for diagnosis. Spongiform change with neuronal loss and gliosis are the crucial changes. Patients usually present with rapidly progressive dementia with myoclonus but CSF examination is required to exclude other infections such as subacute sclerosing panencephalitis.

Iatrogenic Creutzfeldt-Jacob disease may result from surgical transmission such as dural grafting, from administration of pituitary hormones, mainly growth hormone, but is most unlikely from blood products. The aetiology and pathogenesis of this condition is currently the subject of much research. For example, a recent survey has suggested that some general surgical procedures such as hysterectomy are statistically linked with the development of CJD[41], but this remains to be confirmed elsewhere and many questions persist.

Patients with suspected vCJD or other forms of transmissible spongiform encephalopathies may be admitted to the ICU for ventilation or until the diagnosis is confirmed. As far as the authors are aware, the aetiological agents are not acquired during normal clinical care but those surgical instruments in contact with potentially infected tissue should either be disposed of or autoclaved repeatedly at high temperature. Close liaison with the infection control team and the sterile services supply department is mandatory.

Guillian–Barré syndrome

Patients with this condition, the most common cause of neuromuscular paralysis, often require intensive care for prolonged periods for ventilatory support due to respiratory muscle weakness. The pathogenesis is not fully understood but recent studies have suggested an association with *Campylobacter jejuni* infection. Patients with Guillain–Barré syndrome are more likely to have had a recent diarrhoea-like illness, to have *C. jejuni* recovered from their faeces and to have an antibody response to this bacterium[42]. However, by the time the diagnosis is made diarrhoea is often absent or the patient may not even recollect what may have been minor symptoms at the time, and stool cultures are usually negative. It is not believed that the bacterium directly causes this condition but rather that there is cross-reaction between neural and bacterial antigens.

The management of patients with Guillain–Barré syndrome involves ventilation and measures to prevent infection and the other complications of prolonged intensive care. Antibacterial chemotherapy against *C. jejuni* is not indicated as the gastrointestinal infection has usually resolved and there is no evidence that this improves prognosis. The administration of human immunoglobulin is as effective as plasmapheresis in improving outcome by shortening the time on a ventilator[43].

Key points

- Bacterial meningitis is a major cause of morbidity and mortality.
- Empirical antibiotic treatment for bacterial meningitis should start immediately, often before all specimens have been taken and before confirmation of microbiological culture and sensitivity.
- Increased prevalence of antibiotic-resistant organisms will modify the approach to empirical antibiotic therapy.
- Molecular diagnosis is significantly improving the microbiological diagnosis of encephalitis and enhancing our understanding of its aetiology.
- Cerebral abscess should be treated with a combination of drainage of pus and antimicrobial therapy based on sensitivity results.
- *C. botulinum* neurotoxin is the most potent lethal substance known.
- There is an association between Guillain–Barré syndrome and preceding *Campylobacter jejuni* infection.

REFERENCES

1. Connelly M, Noah N (1997) *Surveillance of Bacterial Meningitis in Europe 1996*. Furnival Press, London.
2. Schuchat A, Robinson K, Wenger JD *et al.* (1997) Bacterial meningitis in the United States in 1995. *New England Journal of Medicine* **337**: 970–976.
3. Waage A, Halstensen A, Espevic T (1987) Association between tumour necrosis factor in serum and fatal outcome in patients with meningococcal disease. *Lancet* **i**: 355–357.
4. Pfister HW, Sceld WM (1997) Brain injury in bacterial meningitis: therapeutic implications. *Current Opinion in Neurology* **10**: 254–259.

5. Du Plessis M, Smith AM, Klugman KP (1998) Rapid detection of penicillin resistant *Streptococcus pneumoniae* in cerebrospinal fluid by a semi-nested PCR strategy. *Journal of Clinical Microbiology* **36**: 453–457.
6. Quagliarello V, Scheld WM (1997) Treatment of bacterial meningitis. *New England Journal of Medicine* **336**: 708–716.
7. Scheld WM, Bradley JS (1997) The challenge of penicillin-resistant *Streptococcus pneumoniae* meningitis: current antibiotic therapy in the 1990s. *Clinical Infectious Diseases* **24** (Suppl 2): S213–S221.
8. Morley SL, Levin M (1998) Bacterial meningitis. *Prescribers' Journal* **38**: 129–141.
9. Paris MM, Ramilo O, McCracken GH Jr (1995) Management of meningitis caused by penicillin-resistant *Streptococcus pneumoniae*. *Antimicrobial Agents and Chemotherapy* **39**: 2171–2175.
10. Jones EM, MacGowan AP (1995) Chemotherapy of human infection due to *Listeria monocytogenes*. *European Journal of Clinical Microbiology and Infectious Diseases* **14**: 154–175.
11. Quagliarello V, Scheld WM (1992) Bacterial meningitis: pathogenesis, pathophysiology and progress. *New England Journal of Medicine* **327**: 864–872.
12. McIntyre P, Berkey C, King S et al. (1997) Dexamethasone therapy in bacterial meningitis: a meta-analysis of randomized clinical trials since 1988. *Journal of the American Medical Association* **278**: 925–931.
13. Tauber MG (1998) Management of bacterial meningitis in adults. *Current Opinion in Critical Care* **4**: 276–281.
14. Ramsay M, Kaczmarski E, Rush M et al. (1997) Changing patterns of case ascertainment and trends in meningococcal disease in England and Wales. *Communicable Disease Report (CDR Review)* **7**: R49–R54.
15. Hodgetts TJ, Brett A, Castle N (1998) The early management of meningococcal disease. *Journal of Accident and Emergency Medicine* **15**: 72–76.
16. Milhaud D, Bernardin G, Rastello M et al. (1996) Meningities bacteriennes de l'adulte en reanimation medicale: analyse clinique et étude des facteurs pronostiques. *Presse Medicale* **25**: 353–359.
17. Drake JM, Kulkarni AV (1993) Cerebrospinal fluid shunt infections. *Neurosurgery Quarterly* **3**: 283–294.
18. Working Party on the Use of Antibiotics in Neurosurgery of the British Society for Antimicrobial Chemotherapy (1995) Treatment of infections associated with shunting for hydrocephalus. *British Journal of Hospital Medicine* **53**: 368–373.
19. Infection in Neurosurgery Working Party of the British Society of Antimicrobial Chemotherapy (1994) Antimicrobial prophylaxis in neurosurgery and after head injury. *Lancet* **344**: 1547–1551.
20. Department of Health, Welsh Office, Scottish Office, Department of Health and the Department of Health and Social Services (Northern Ireland) (1996) *Immunisation against Infectious Diseases*. HMSO, London.
21. Johnson RT (1995) Acute encephalitis. *Clinical Infectious Diseases* **23**: 219–226.
22. Marton R, Gotlieb-Steimatsky T, Klein C et al. (1996) Acute herpes simplex encephalitis: clinical assessment and prognostic data. *Acta Neurologica Scandinavica* **93**: 149–155.
23. Tang Y-W, Mitchell PS, Espy MJ et al. (1999) Molecular diagnosis of herpes simplex virus infections in the central nervous system. *Journal of Clinical Microbiology* **37**: 2127–2136.

24. Read SJ, Kurtz JB (1999) Laboratory diagnosis of common viral infections of the central nervous system by using a single multiplex PCR screening assay. *Journal of Clinical Microbiology* **37**: 1352–1355.
25. Klapper PE, Cleator GM (1998) European guidelines for the diagnosis and management of patients with herpes simplex encephalitis. *Clinical Microbiology and Infection* **4**: 178–180.
26. Lipkin WI (1997) European consensus on viral encephalitis. *Lancet* **349**: 299–300.
27. Hagensee ME, Bauwens JE, Kjos B *et al.* (1994) Brain abscess following marrow transplantation: experience at the Fred Hutchinson Cancer Research Centre, 1984–1992. *Clinical Infectious Diseases* **19**: 402–428.
28. Levy RM (1994) Brain abscess and subdural empyema. *Current Opinion in Neurology* **7**: 223–228.
29. Mamelak AN, Mampalan TJ, Obana WG *et al.* (1995) Improved management of multiple brain abscesses: a combined surgical and medical approach. *Neurosurgery* **36**: 76–85.
30. Shapiro RL, Hatheway C, Swerdlow DL (1998) Botulism in the United States: a clinical and epidemiological review. *Annals of Internal Medicine* **129**: 221–228.
31. Therre H (1999) Botulism in the European Union. *Eurosurveillance* **4**: 1–12.
32. Bruno S (1998) Botulism caused by Italian bottled vegetables. *Lancet* **352**: 884.
33. Willatts SM, Winter RJ (1992) *Principles and Protocols in Intensive Care*, pp 237–241. Farrand Press, London.
34. Gergen PJ, McQuillan GM, Kiely M *et al.* (1995) A population-based serological survey of immunity to tetanus in the United States. *New England Journal of Medicine* **332**: 761–766.
35. Bardenheier B, Prevots DR, Khetsuriani N *et al.* (1998) Tetanus surveillance – United States, 1995–1997. *MMWR CDC Surveillance Summaries* **47**: 1–13.
36. Sanford JP (1995) Tetanus – forgotten but not gone. *New England Journal of Medicine* **332**: 813–814.
37. Camacho JA, Jimenez JM, Diaz A *et al.* (1997) Severe-grade tetanus in a multipurpose ICU: review of 13 cases. *Enfermedades Infecciosas y Microbiologia Clinica* **15**: 243–245.
38. Johnson TJ, Gibbs CJ (1998) Creutzfeldt–Jakob disease and other transmissible spongiform encephalopathies. *New England Journal of Medicine* **339**: 1994–2004.
39. Haywood AM (1997) Transmissible spongiform encephalopathies. *New England Journal of Medicine* **337**: 1821–1828.
40. Petersen RB (1999) Antemortem diagnosis of variant Creutzfeldt–Jakob disease. *Lancet* **353**: 163–164.
41. Collins S, Law MG, Fletcher A *et al.* (1999) Surgical treatment and risk of sporadic Creutzfeldt–Jakob disease: a case control study. *Lancet* **353**: 693–697.
42. Rees JH, Soudain SE, Gregson NA *et al.* (1995) *Campylobacter jejuni* infection and Guillain–Barré syndrome. *New England Journal of Medicine* **333**: 1374–1379.
43. Van der Meche FGA, Schmitz PIM and the Dutch Guillian–Barré Study Group (1992) A randomized trial comparing intravenous immunoglobulin and plasma exchange in Guillian–Barré syndrome. *New England Journal of Medical* **326**: 1123–1129.

12 Infection in immunosuppressed patients

Patients with underlying malignancy, patients on chemotherapy, steroids or other immunosuppressive agents, human immunodeficiency virus (HIV)-positive patients and patients following bone marrow or solid organ transplantation are very susceptible to infection, especially to opportunist infections. However, the term 'immunosuppressed patient' also includes many patients admitted to the intensive care unit (ICU) following multiple trauma or major surgery but in these patients it is usually not clinically evident. As the prognosis following treatment of many malignancies improves and as the number and complexity of solid organ transplantation (e.g. pancreas, bowel) increases, the need for temporary organ support or for the management of infection in the ICU is likely to become more common. Consequently, some understanding of the complex issues involved in the diagnosis and management of infection in immunosuppressed patients is required, especially in those hospitals with haematology/oncology units or with transplantation programmes.

Many of these patients may be on antibiotic prophylaxis to minimize the risk of primary infection, relapse or recurrence of infection, such as co-trimoxazole to prevent *Pneumocystis carinii* pneumonia, fluconazole to prevent cryptococcal meningitis, ciprofloxacin to decontaminate the bowel in patients undergoing bone marrow transplantation and aciclovir to prevent herpes infection. Such prophylaxis must be considered when assessing the aetiology and source of infection and may explain negative laboratory investigations. Furthermore, a knowledge of the patient's prophylactic regimen may influence initial empirical antimicrobial chemotherapy in the patient with suspected infection, since resistant organisms are more likely in patients who have been on long-term prophylaxis. Therefore, while common pathogens such as *Streptococcus pneumoniae* and *Escherichia coli* remain important causes of infection, these pathogens may be more antibiotic resistant than those from non-immunosuppressed patients and the range of pathogens that must be considered is wider.

PATIENT CATEGORIES AND RISK FACTORS

Certain infections are more likely in particular patient risk groups and are more likely to occur at certain times. An understanding of this assists in prioritizing investigations and in deciding empirical therapy.

Solid organ transplantation

Many bacteria, viruses, fungi and parasites are capable of causing infection in solid organ transplant recipients and the risk and cause of infection are greatly influenced by the immunosuppressive agents used. For example, prednisone impairs lymphocyte and macrophage function, azathioprine inhibits cell proliferation by interfering with DNA synthesis, and cyclosporin blocks T cell activation[1]. Leukopenia or neutropenia due to immunosuppressive agents such as azathioprine, and bone marrow suppression arising from infection with cytomegalovirus (CMV), may also occur following solid organ transplantation. During the first month following solid organ transplantation, most infections are related to the surgical procedure and may reflect technical difficulties at the time of the procedure, e.g. ascending cholangitis due to biliary stricture after liver transplantation, or mediastinitis following heart transplantation. Infections occurring during this period are usually bacterial but reactivation of herpes simplex virus infections is not uncommon. From 2 to 6 months following transplantation, opportunist pathogens such as *P. carinii*, *Aspergillus* spp. and *Toxoplasma gondii* are more prevalent. Reactivation of previous infection with *Mycobacterium tuberculosis* and CMV may also occur at this time, and from 6 months onwards CMV and varicella-zoster virus (VZV) infections become more likely even though the overall incidence of infection falls.

Pneumonia is amongst the most important infections and is relatively common after heart transplantation (Table 12.1) when both *P. carinii* and *Legionella* spp. should be considered as possible causes[2]. Following liver transplantation, gut-derived organisms such as enterococci and aerobic Gram-negative bacilli are important causes of infection and 90% of fungal infections occur within the first 2 months after surgery[3]. The transplant procedure, the interval following surgery and the results of pretransplant screening, e.g. positive

Table 12.1 Infections following heart transplantation.

Time[a]	Infection	Pathogens[b]
Early (<2 months)	Pneumonia	*S. pneumoniae*, nosocomial bacteria (e.g. *Pseudomonas*)
	Sternal wound infections	Staphylococci, Gram-negative bacilli, *Candida* spp.
	CNS	*T. gondii*, fungal brain abscesses
Later (>2 months)	Pneumonia	*P. carinii*, CMV, *Nocardia asteroides*
	CNS	*Listeria* meningoencephalitis, *Cryptococcus* meningitis, JC virus
	Skin	Reactivation of VZV

[a] Following transplant.
[b] CMV, cytomegalovirus; VZV, varicella-zoster virus; CNS, central nervous system.

serology for CMV or VZV, should all be considered when assessing the likely cause of infection.

Bone marrow transplantation

Bone marrow transplantation, especially autologous bone marrow transplantation (i.e. where the recipient serves as the donor), is increasingly used in the management of malignant and non-malignant haematological diseases as, amongst other things, the risk of infection is less than that following allogeneic transplantation. During the early post-transplantation period, profound neutropenia and a state of combined cell-mediated and humoral immune deficiency exists. This partly recovers but phagocyte function, T cell immune function and immunoglobulin production may be defective for a year or more following transplantation[4]. For allogenic recipients, the degree of histocompatibility mismatch, the use of related versus unrelated donors, the bone marrow transplantation conditioning regimen and the presence and treatment of graft-versus-host disease all influence the risk, cause and presentation of infection. As with solid organ transplants, the aetiology of infection is influenced by the interval post-transplantation[4, 5] as follows.

First month

This is a period during which granulocytopenia, damaged mucosal surfaces due to chemotherapy and radiation, predispose to infection. Bacteraemia and bacterial soft tissue or respiratory tract infections are most common; reactivated herpes simplex viral infections are now less common due to the widespread use of aciclovir prophylaxis. Before the widespread use of prophylaxis with fluoroquinolones, bacteraemia caused by Gram-negative bacilli such as *Pseudomonas aeruginosa* was more common than Gram-positive infection but this is no longer the case; the mortality rate from Gram-positive infection is, however, lower at approximately 5%[5].

Second to third month

This period is characterized by cellular immune deficiency and subnormal antibody responses, and these immune deficiencies are more severe and more persistent in patients with graft-versus-host disease. Pulmonary aspergillosis, candidiasis and CMV infection (e.g. pneumonitis and colitis) may be seen at this time; *P. carinii* is now less common following the use of widespread prophylaxis with co-trimoxazole.

Third month onwards

Recovery of humoral and cellular immunity occurs, and VZV is the single most common infection. VZV infection may be severe with hepatitis or encephalitis and may be complicated by secondary bacterial skin infection (e.g. cellulitis) or pneumonia[6].

195

Human immunodeficiency virus

The improved outcome from HIV infection due to combined anti-retroviral therapy and the use of prophylactic antimicrobial agents to prevent opportunist infections has changed the incidence and range of infections seen in patients with HIV. The patient population (i.e. whether intravenous drug users, homosexuals, etc.) influences the category of infection seen; sexually transmitted diseases such as genital herpes are more likely in homosexuals, whereas staphylococcal or fungal endocarditis is associated with intravenous drug users. The risk of infection increases as the CD4$^+$ count declines to less than 300 μl^{-1}, and the most prevalent infections are *Candida* oesophagitis, *P. carinii* pneumonia, *Mycobacterium avium* complex bacteraemia and CMV[7]. The increasing use of antimicrobial prophylaxis has resulted recently in a decline in the incidence of cryptococcal meningitis (fluconazole), *M. avium* complex disease (rifabutin) and secondary *P. carinii* pneumonia (co-trimoxazole), but the incidence of toxoplasmosis has not changed[7]. Furthermore, the use of highly active anti-retroviral therapy (HAART) in the last few years has resulted in improvements in the resolution of opportunist infections and a fundamental change in the natural history of HIV disease[8]. Respiratory tract infections are especially common; bacterial pneumonia such as that caused by *S. pneumoniae* may be accompanied by bacteraemia. *P. carinii*, tuberculosis and fungal pneumonia, e.g. *Aspergillus* spp., *Cryptococcus* spp. and *Histoplasma* spp. (uncommon in Europe), should also be considered in the HIV-positive patient with pulmonary symptoms. In the patient with advanced HIV disease, non-specific features such as fever, weight loss and fatigue may suggest tuberculosis as cavitation is unusual and the chest X-ray may be normal[9]. Finally, Kaposi's sarcoma, lymphomas and non-specific or lymphoid interstitial pneumonitis may present like infection and therefore should also be considered in the differential diagnosis of respiratory infection in patients with HIV.

DIAGNOSTIC AND MANAGEMENT ASPECTS

Comprehensive clinical assessment such as regular examinations of the mouth, chest, abdomen, intravascular line sites and perineum, followed by sensible use of appropriate investigations, are the initial key components in the effective management of the immunosuppressed patient with infection. A knowledge of the nature of the immune deficiency and the likely causative pathogens should prompt relevant investigations and the commencement of appropriate empirical antimicrobial chemotherapy. However, the management of infection in these patients is greatly helped by a multidisciplinary team approach involving oncologists, haematologists, respiratory physicians, radiologists, surgeons, infectious disease physicians, microbiologists/virologists and others. For example, consultation with a respiratory physician and radiologist in the management of the patient with lung infection of unknown aetiology may ensure that the laboratory receives those specimens most likely to confirm a microbiological diagnosis. Repeat diagnostic procedures such as bronchoscopy may not be possible because of the severity of illness (e.g. haemorrhage due to thrombo-cytopenia) and consequently early diagnosis and appropriate initial management are essential. A consideration of all the possible clinical illnesses that the immunosuppressed patient requiring ICU care may develop is beyond the scope of this book, but those discussed below are amongst the more common or important.

Pyrexia in the neutropenic patient

Neutropenia is most common following bone marrow transplantation or in patients during or following intensive chemotherapy for haematological or solid organ malignancy. The risk of fatal infection increases with the duration (especially if 10 days or greater) and severity of neutropenia, i.e. $<0.1 \times 10^9$ neutrophils l^{-1}. Although significant pyrexia (i.e. $>39°C$ on one occasion or $38.5°C$ on two occasions) may be due to the disease process itself, or administration of antineoplastic agents or blood products, infection is the commonest cause, but in up to 50% of patients no aetiological agent is ever confirmed. The routine use of surveillance cultures, e.g. weekly or bi-weekly nose, throat, urine and stool cultures, is of questionable value unless resistant organisms are locally prevalent, as is locating the patient in protective isolation in a laminar airflow unit following bone marrow transplantation, which is the practice in many centres. The results of surveillance and other cultures together with baseline serology for certain viruses (e.g. CMV) should be reviewed in the febrile neutropenic patient. For example, recent colonization with *Candida tropicalis* or *C. kruseii* is more likely to predict infection, unlike *C. albicans* when colonization without infection is quite common[10]. Relevant investigations which should be considered are outlined in Table 12.2.

As many patients may be, or have recently been, on antibacterial agents, repeat blood cultures are required. The greater the volume of blood cultured, the higher the yield for the detection of candidaemia; culturing 20 ml significantly increases the yield compared with 10 ml[11]. Other specimens may be indicated depending on symptoms or signs, e.g. faeces should be taken for microscopy, culture and analysis for *Clostridium difficile* toxin, if diarrhoea is present, or if there has been a change in bowel habit. Tissue biopsy under ultrasound or computerized tomography (CT) guidance, or even during surgery, may be required if initial investigations are suggestive of infection.

To date, the measurement of acute-phase reactants such as C-reactive protein and cytokines such as interleukin 6 have been disappointing in specifically diagnosing infection. However, repeated measurements over time may strongly indicate the presence of an infection[10] but further research is needed to clarify the role of routinely monitoring cytokine levels. Haematopoietic growth factors such as granulocyte colony-stimulating factor are increasingly used to shorten the duration of neutropenia, but these should only be prescribed by a haematologist or oncologist and should be reserved for situations where the neutrophil count is expected to remain below $0.1 \times 10^9 l^{-1}$ for many days[12]. Granulocyte–macrophage colony-stimulating factor may be more logical in the presence of fungal infection but its effectiveness remains unproven.

Table 12.2 Investigations in the febrile neutropenic patient.

Investigation	Test	Comment
Microbiology	Blood cultures	At least two sets, including one or more through a central intravascular line if possible
	Urine culture	Systemic yeast infection may be indicated by positive urine culture
	Respiratory	BAL or PBS rather than sputum is more likely to yield a fungal or viral aetiology
	Skin biopsy	Rash may indicate systemic *Candida* or cryptococcal infection
	Cerebrospinal fluid	As clinically indicated
	Serology	Compare with baseline results but may not get seroconversion due to immunosuppression
Imaging	Chest X-ray	May be negative or non-specific; compare with earlier images
	Sinus X-rays	Symptoms (e.g. pain, epistaxis) may indicate *Aspergillus* or *Mucor* infections
	CT scan	'Air crescent' sign in CT of chest is very suggestive of pulmonary aspergillosis and spiral CT is useful in suspected fungal infection

BAL, bronchoalveolar lavage; PBS, protected brush specimen; CT, computed tomography.

The approach to the treatment of fever of unknown aetiology in the neutropenic patient is usually to start empirical treatment with broad-spectrum antibacterial agents once appropriate specimens have been taken. There has been considerable debate in recent years over the relative merits of monotherapy compared with a β-lactam plus aminoglycoside combination. Many now consider that treatment with a single broad-spectrum agent such as a carbapenem (imipenem or meropenem) or a cephalosporin with antipseudomonal activity (ceftazidime) or a penicillin (piperacillin plus tazobactam) is adequate for most patients[5, 13], and furthermore monotherapy reduces the risk of side-effects such as renal toxicity that may follow the use of aminoglycosides. However, an aminoglycoside is indicated if the patient is acutely ill, e.g. septic shock, or if there is evidence of infection with *P. aeruginosa* or multi-resistant Gram-negative bacilli such as *Serratia* spp. (if sensitive *in vitro*). Despite the increasing prevalence of bacteraemia caused by Gram-positive bacteria such as *Staphylococcus epidermidis* or *Enterococcus faecalis*, a glycopeptide is usually not indicated as part of the initial regimen unless an intravascular line infection is strongly suspected. If there is no response to treatment within 24–48 hours, an aminoglycoside and/or a glycopeptide should be added to the initial regimen. Systemic antifungal therapy is indicated if one or more of the following occur[14]:

1. There is no response to broad-spectrum antibacterial agents after 72–96 hours – 48 hours if prolonged neutropenia, history of *Candida* colonization, clinically suspicious lesions or bone marrow transplant patient.
2. There are new infiltrates on chest X-ray.
3. Fungi are recovered from blood or other normally sterile sites.
4. *C. tropicalis* is isolated from any site.
5. Clinical signs and symptoms (e.g. skin rash) suggestive of fungal infection are present.

Amphotericin B remains the antifungal drug of choice because it is active against *Candida*, *Aspergillus*, *Mucor*, *Cryptococcus*, sporotrichosis and most other fungal pathogens. Lipid-associated preparations such as liposomal amphotericin B (AmBisone) are preferred if renal or other toxicities preclude conventional amphotericin B, or for the treatment of infections where effective concentrations are not achievable with conventional preparations, such as in the treatment of *Mucor* infection[14]. It has recently been demonstrated that liposomal amphotericin B is associated with fewer breakthrough fungal infections and a lower incidence of toxicity when used empirically in the therapy of patients with fever and neutropenia[15]. Triazoles such as fluconazole and itraconazole are not recommended for the empirical treatment of fungal infection in the neutropenic patient as they are not as active and their spectrum of activity is narrower. Where there is evidence of pulmonary infection, the addition of co-trimoxazole to cover *P. carinii* should be considered, especially if the patient is not on prophylaxis (see below). Antiviral chemotherapy is added if there is no response to combined antibacterial and antifungal treatment; aciclovir is the treatment of choice for herpes simplex or varicella-zoster infections, ganciclovir is indicated for diagnosed or suspected CMV infection, and ribavirin administered via a small-particle aerosol generator is suggested for respiratory syncytial virus infections. A suggested approach to the sequential antimicrobial therapy of fever in the neutropenic patient is outlined in Figure 12.1.

Respiratory infections in the immunosuppressed host

A wide range of upper or lower respiratory tract infections caused by common pathogens such as *S. pneumoniae* occur in immunosuppressed patients but these may be more severe than normal and infection may be caused by opportunist pathogens such as *P. carinii* and atypical mycobacteria. Viral infections (i.e. caused by respiratory syncytial virus, influenza, parainfluenza, adenovirus and CMV) are not uncommon; at least 5% or more of all bone marrow transplant patients develop a potentially serious respiratory infection and 10–40% will die following the development of pneumonia[16, 17]. The

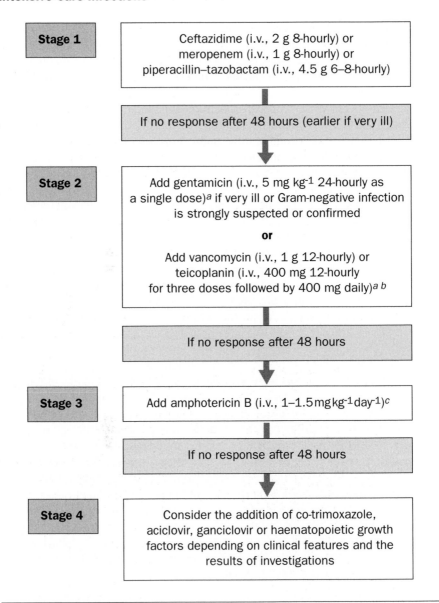

Figure 12.1 items:

Stage 1
Ceftazidime (i.v., 2 g 8-hourly) or meropenem (i.v., 1 g 8-hourly) or piperacillin–tazobactam (i.v., 4.5 g 6–8-hourly)

If no response after 48 hours (earlier if very ill)

Stage 2
Add gentamicin (i.v., 5 mg kg^{-1} 24-hourly as a single dose)[a] if very ill or Gram-negative infection is strongly suspected or confirmed

or

Add vancomycin (i.v., 1 g 12-hourly) or teicoplanin (i.v., 400 mg 12-hourly for three doses followed by 400 mg daily)[a][b]

If no response after 48 hours

Stage 3
Add amphotericin B (i.v., 1–1.5 mg kg^{-1} day^{-1})[c]

If no response after 48 hours

Stage 4
Consider the addition of co-trimoxazole, aciclovir, ganciclovir or haematopoietic growth factors depending on clinical features and the results of investigations

[a] Regular estimation of serum levels should be carried out to minimize toxicity and to optimize dosage.
[b] Vancomycin preferred for suspected staphylococcal infections, teicoplanin preferred for suspected enterococcal infections and in patients with renal impairment or difficult venous access.
[c] Liposomal preparations or other lipid-based preparations may be preferred as discussed in text.

Figure 12.1 Algorithm for the use of antimicrobial agents in the management of the febrile neutropenic patient.

diagnostic approach depends on the severity of infection, the clinical and radiological presentation and the facilities for bronchoscopy. One approach is to consider whether infection is localized or diffuse and to assess the response to initial antibacterial therapy. Infections characterized by localized infiltrates on chest X-ray caused by *Haemophilus influenzae*, *Staphylococcus aureus* or *P. aeruginosa* may be readily diagnosed from sputum and blood cultures, and may respond to broad-spectrum antibiotics. The aetiology of diffuse infiltrates on chest X-ray unresponsive to antibacterial agents may not be confirmed unless bronchoscopy to obtain bronchoalveolar lavage is conducted to exclude *P. carinii*, *Aspergillus* spp., *Legionella* spp., *Mycobacterium* spp., etc.[18]. There is now a wide range of laboratory investigations (Figure 12.2; Plate 12), including direct antigen detection and polymerase chain reaction (PCR)[19], available to maximize the yield from respiratory specimens (see Chapters 4 and 7) which greatly facilitate specific diagnoses (e.g. rapid antigen tests for CMV), and close liaison with the microbiology laboratory is therefore strongly recommended.

Empirical approaches to therapy should involve a logical sequential approach not unlike that for the treatment of fever in the neutropenic patient. However, in the severely ill patient requiring ventilation, it may be necessary to include antibacterial, antifungal and antiviral agents even before all investigations have been carried out. In patients with HIV, *P. carinii* remains the most common

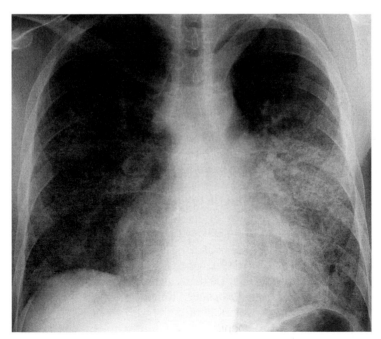

Figure 12.2 Diagnosis of *P. carinii*. Chest X-ray showing 'ground glass' appearance in the right mid-zone characteristic of early *P. carinii* pneumonia. Appearance on the left represents onset of 'fluffy' consolidation usually seen later.

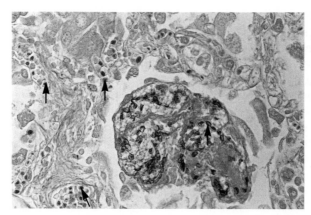

Plate 12 Diagnosis of
P. carinii. Histological
section of lung tissue
(Grocott stain) showing
P. carinii cysts (arrows)
indicative of infection.

serious opportunistic infection. The differential diagnosis in the bone marrow transplant patient or the patient on chemotherapy includes acute lung injury secondary to radiation or chemotherapy, and diffuse alveolar haemorrhage. Co-trimoxazole (either i.v. or oral, 120 mg kg^{-1} per day in two to four divided doses for 21 days) is the treatment of choice[20]. Alternative regimens include clindamycin–primaquine, pentamidine or atovaquone. Chemoprophylaxis following recovery is usually indicated for patients with a CD4$^+$ lymphocyte count below 200 µl^{-1}. Further details on antifungal and antiviral agents used in immuno-suppressed patients are outlined in Table 12.3.

Intracranial infections

Symptoms such as fever, headache and confusion, or coma should suggest central nervous infection. Whilst conventional causes of meningitis and encephalitis (see Chapter 11), intracranial haemorrhage or malignancy may be responsible, opportunist infections such as toxoplasmosis, CMV and *Cryptococcus* should be considered. Diagnosis is dependent on a combination of microbiological examination of the cerebrospinal fluid (CSF) and imaging of the central nervous system (CNS) such as CT scanning.

Infection due to *T. gondii* is a well-recognized complication of acquired immune deficiency syndrome (AIDS) and should always be considered in a HIV-positive patient with encephalitis and intracerebral lesion seen on CT or magnetic resonance imaging (MRI). Clinical features include headache, confusion and fever but the CSF may be unremarkable. Serum may be negative but the CSF is usually positive for *Toxoplasma* antibodies. CT or MRI reveals one or more enhancing lesions in over 90% of patients[21]. Toxic side-effects such as vomiting, diarrhoea and leukopenia arising from treatment with pyrimethamine and sulfadiazine are relatively common but relapse occurs in most patients if therapy is stopped. A severely depressed level of consciousness at presentation, a history of Kaposi's sarcoma and the presence of other opportunist infections such as *P. carini* are associated with a poor prognosis[21]. Pyrimethamine (orally,

Table 12.3 Antifungal (excluding pneumocystis infection) and antiviral agents that may be used to treat lower respiratory infections in the immunosuppressed patient (based on references 13 and 14).

Class of agent	Agent	Comment
Antifungal	Amphotericin B, $1–1.5\,mg\,kg^{-1}\,day^{-1}$	Smaller doses ($0.7\,mg\,kg^{-1}$) may be sufficient to treat yeast infections[a]
	Liposomal or lipid-associated amphotericin B, $3\,mg\,kg^{-1}\,day^{-1}$ or more	Drug of choice for *Mucor* and *Fusarium* spp.[a]
	Fluconazole $400\,mg\,kg^{-1}\,day^{-1}$ or more	Inactive against *Aspergillus*. Alternative to amphotericin B for *Candida* and *Cryptococcus* (with flucytosine) infections
	Itraconazole $200–400\,mg\,day^{-1}$	Alternative to amphotericin B to treat invasive aspergillosis
Antiviral	Aciclovir, i.v., $5–10\,mg\,kg^{-1}$ 8-hourly for at least 7 days	Treatment of choice for herpes simplex; also used to treat varicella-zoster ($10\,mg\,kg^{-1}$ t.d.s.) infection
	Ganciclovir, $5–6\,mg\,kg^{-1}$ 12-hourly	Neutropenia is the main toxic side-effect
	Foscarnet, $40–60\,mg\,kg^{-1}$ t.d.s.	Renal toxicity possible especially if the patient is also on cyclosporin A
	Tribavirin by aerosol $20\,mg\,ml^{-1}$ of water over 18–20 hours per day	Believed to be of some benefit for respiratory syncytial virus but not proven in clinical trials

[a] Test dose usually recommended.

200 mg load, then $75\,mg\,day^{-1}$) with sulfadiazine (orally, $25\,mg\,kg^{-1}$ up to 2 g 6-hourly) remains the treatment of choice but side-effects may necessitate changing to alternative regimens, which include clindamycin plus pyrimethamine, atovaquone and newer macrolides with pyrimethamine[22]. The high relapse rate of approximately 50% necessitates anti-*Toxoplasma* treatment for life.

The clinical manifestations of CMV infection in the immunosuppressed patient are very varied and include pneumonia, hepatitis, colitis, a non-specific febrile illness, leukopenia or thrombocytopenia, retinitis and encephalitis. Infection should be suspected in seropositive transplant recipients or seronegative transplant patients who have received a seropositive organ or seropositive blood products. CMV encephalitis is characterized by fever, confusion, coma, behavioural changes, ataxia and focal neurological signs such as limb weakness[23]. Most patients have infection in another organ or system but this may not be clinically evident and may be confirmed only with histology or at autopsy. Viral culture of the CSF is usually negative and the reliability of differential CSF : serum antibodies to CMV has not been validated. PCR on the CSF is increasingly used and offers the potential advantage of a speedy diagnosis. However, given the underlying illness and general health of many patients with this infection, the prognosis is poor despite the use of antiviral therapy such as ganciclovir, and the median survival is only 42 days from the onset of symptoms[23]. Preventive strategies include the use of CMV-negative organs or CMV-negative or leuko-depleted blood products in seronegative patients, long-term prophylaxis with aciclovir or ganciclovir, and hyperimmune or standard intravenous immune globulin[24]. Ganciclovir prophylaxis (i.v., $5 \, mg \, kg^{-1}$ 12-hourly), which has better anti-CMV activity than aciclovir, is probably the best option for high-risk patients such as lung transplant recipients and possibly allogeneic bone marrow transplant recipients. Pre-emptive therapy with ganciclovir following rapid diagnosis is advised for lower-risk patients such as seropositive patients undergoing renal, liver or heart transplantation[24].

Meningitis in patients with HIV infection or in other patients with cell-mediated immunodeficiency may be due to *Cryptococcus neoformans* but common causes in the general population such as *Neisseria meningitidis* or enteroviruses (see Chapter 4) should not be dismissed as unlikely. Additional laboratory processing of CSF samples (see Chapters 4 and 11) is, however, required to ensure that a diagnosis of cryptococcal meningitis is not missed. CSF microscopy, including Indian ink stains to detect capsulated yeasts and cryptococcal antigen detection in the CSF and serum, will improve the rate of a positive diagnosis. Sequential titres of the CSF antigen load have been shown to predict outcome; 83% of 73 patients with AIDS who ultimately responded to therapy showed a decrease in CSF titre during treatment but serum titres were not predictive of relapse[25]. The treatment of choice is a combination of amphotericin B (i.v., 0.7 mg or higher each day) plus flucytosine (i.v., $75–100 \, mg \, kg^{-1}$ each day)[13]. Flucytosine is, however, toxic to the bone marrow and weekly serum assays of blood levels are required. Combination therapy should be continued for 2 weeks and should be followed by oral fluconazole or oral itraconazole for some weeks afterwards to prevent relapse.

Key points

- Infection is more common and more severe in immunosuppressed patients and may be caused by both conventional and opportunist pathogens.
- Neutropenic sepsis is a medical emergency and rapid progression to death may occur within hours.
- The successful management of infection is very much dependent on a coordinated multidisciplinary approach.
- An understanding of the underlying condition of the patient is essential in assessing which infections are most likely and when.
- A sequential approach to the antimicrobial treatment of fever in the neutropenic patient involving antibacterial, antifungal and antiviral agents is recommended.
- Good specimens such as bronchoalveolar lavage or protected brush specimens are important in confirming the aetiology of lower respiratory tract infections.
- Analysis of CSF specimens and good diagnostic imaging are the mainstays of diagnosis in CNS infections such as toxoplasmosis and cryptococcal meningitis.

REFERENCES

1. Patel R, Paya CV (1997) Infections in solid-organ transplant recipients. *Clinical Microbiology Reviews* **10**: 86–124.
2. Petri WA Jr (1994) Infections in heart transplant recipients. *Clinical Infectious Diseases* **18**: 141–148.
3. Winston DJ, Emmanouilides C, Busuttil RW (1995) Infections in liver transplant recipients. *Clinical Infectious Diseases* **21**: 1077–1091.
4. LaRocco MT, Burgert SJ (1997) Infection in the bone marrow transplant recipient and role of the microbiology laboratory in clinical transplantation. *Clinical Microbiology Reviews* **10**: 277–297.
5. Winston DJ (1995) Prophylaxis and treatment of infection in the bone marrow transplant recipient. In: *Current Clinical Topics in Infectious Diseases* (eds Remington JS, Swartz MN), pp 293–321. Blackwell Scientific, Oxford.
6. Cohen JI, Brunell PA, Straus PE *et al.* (1999) Recent advances in varicella zoster infection. *Annals of Internal Medicine* **130**: 922–932.
7. Moore RD, Chaisson RE (1996) Natural history of opportunistic disease in an HIV-infected urban clinical cohort. *Annals of Internal Medicine* **124**: 633–642.
8. Sepkowitz KA (1998) Effect of HAART on natural history of AIDS-related opportunistic disorders. *Lancet* **351**: 228–230.
9. Miller R (1996) HIV-associated respiratory diseases. *Lancet* **348**: 307–312.
10. Gillespie T, Masterson RG (1998) Investigation of infection in the neutropenic patient with fever. *Journal of Hospital Infection* **38**: 77–91.

11. Denning DW, Evans EGV, Kibbler CC *et al.* (1997) Guidelines for the investigation of invasive fungal infections in haematological malignancy and solid organ transplantation. *European Journal of Clinical Microbiology and Infectious Diseases* **16**: 424–436.

12. Hussein AM, Elkordy M, Peters WP (1996) The use of growth factors with antibiotics in the setting of neutropenic fever. *American Journal of Medicine* **100**: 15–16.

13. Kibbler CC (1995) Neutropenic infections; strategies for empirical therapy. *Journal of Hospital Infection* **36** (Suppl B): 107–117.

14. Working Party of the British Society for Antimicrobial Chemotherapy (1997) Therapy of deep fungal infection in haematological malignancy. *Journal of Antimicrobial Chemotherapy* **40**: 779–788.

15. Walsh TJ, Finberg RW, Arndt C *et al.* (1999) Liposomal amphotericin B for empirical therapy in patients with persistent fever and neutropenia. *New England Journal of Medicine* **340**: 764–771.

16. Wood MJ (1998) Viral infections in neutropenia – current problems and chemotherapeutic control. *Journal of Antimicrobial Chemotherapy* **41** (Suppl D): 81–93.

17. Muir D, Pillay D (1998) Respiratory virus infections in immunocompromised patients. *Journal of Medical Microbiology* **47**: 561–562.

18. Mulinde J, Joshi M (1998) The diagnosis and therapeutic approach to lower respiratory tract infections in the neutropenic patient. *Journal of Antimicrobial Chemotherapy* **41** (Suppl D): 51–55.

19. Thompson RB Jr (1999) Laboratory diagnosis of respiratory infections. *Current Opinion in Infectious Diseases* **12**: 115–119.

20. Morris-Jones SD, Easterbrook PJ (1997) Current issues in the treatment and prophylaxis of *Pneumocystis carinii* pneumonia in HIV infection. *Journal of Antimicrobial Chemotherapy* **40**: 315–318.

21. Porter SB, Sande MA (1992) Toxoplasmosis of the central nervous system in the acquired immunodeficiency syndrome. *New England Journal of Medicine* **327**: 1643–1648.

22. Lane HC, Laughton BE, Fallon J *et al.* (1994) Recent advances in the management of AIDS-related opportunistic infections. *Annals of Internal Medicine* **120**: 945–955.

23. Arribas JR, Storch GA, Clifford DB *et al.* (1996) Cytomegalovirus encephalitis. *Annals of Internal Medicine* **125**: 577–587.

24. Winston DJ (1995) Prevention of cytomegalovirus diseases in transplant recipients. *Lancet* **346**: 1380–1381.

25. Powderly WG, Cloud GA, Dismukes WE *et al.* (1994) Measurement of cryptococcal antigen in serum and cerebrospinal fluid: value in the management of AIDS-associated cryptococcal meningitis. *Clinical Infectious Diseases* **18**: 789–792.

13 Infections of the cardiovascular system

Infections of the cardiovascular system in the intensive care unit (ICU) are not as common as those of the lower respiratory tract but they are important because they may be life threatening (e.g. mycotic aneurysm), treatment is often complex and infection may result in considerable morbidity. The majority of patients with infections not associated with surgery, e.g. infective endocarditis, are often diagnosed and treated on a general medical ward or in a coronary care unit. Many patients following vascular surgery are admitted to the ICU for observation and organ support during the immediate postoperative period, and postoperative cardiac surgery patients may be cared for in a specialist high-dependency unit or designated cardiac surgery ICU, and consequently infections in this last group may not be frequently encountered in the general ICU. All patients with cardiovascular infections, whether requiring ICU care or otherwise, should be cared for in conjunction with relevant specialists, i.e. cardiac or vascular surgeon, cardiologist, and microbiologist or infectious disease physician. The presentation, diagnosis and treatment of patients with prosthetic infections (i.e. heart valve, aortic or peripheral vascular graft) are not straightforward and suboptimal care can have devastating consequences. The most convenient classification of cardiovascular infections is medical or surgical, but some infections, e.g. prosthetic valve infective endocarditis, may straddle both categories.

NON-SURGICAL INFECTIONS

Infective endocarditis

Although relatively uncommon, a missed diagnosis of infective endocarditis has potentially fatal complications. Involvement of one or more valves, i.e. valvular endocarditis, is more common than mural endocarditis but the presentation, diagnosis and management of the latter are similar[1]. Apart from patients with prosthetic valves, streptococcal endocarditis is still more common than staphylococcal endocarditis but infection with other organisms such as *Aspergillus* spp. after valve replacement, or *Haemophilus* spp., must also be considered. Increasingly in France and elsewhere, endocarditis caused by *Bartonella* spp., fastidious Gram-negative bacteria responsible for trench fever, cat scratch disease and bacillary angiomatosis, is being described in homeless people[2]. Laboratory confirmation is not, however, straightforward and these bacteria may therefore be responsible for some cases of 'culture-negative' endocarditis. In addition, consideration of antimicrobial prophylaxis in those patients at risk is important in every ICU.

Presentation

Infective endocarditis should be considered in the differential diagnosis of any patient with fever and a heart murmur, especially a new murmur, or one that has changed recently in character. The terms 'subacute' and 'acute' are now less relevant than previously, when diagnosis was often delayed, and the classification is now based on the aetiology, e.g. staphylococcal, streptococcal, etc. Confirming a diagnosis in many patients may be not always be straight-forward as the presenting features of fever, an unexplained embolic phenomenon, or rapidly deteriorating cardiac failure are relatively non-specific and may be due to a number of other disease processes.

Diagnosis

Recently proposed guidelines for making a diagnosis, i.e. the Duke criteria, have been shown to be highly specific in ruling out infective endocarditis and are superior to previous criteria[3, 4]. These criteria emphasize clinical features, repeat positive blood cultures and echocardiography, especially transoesophageal echocardiography (TOE), which is more sensitive than transthoracic echocardio-graphy (TTE) but is not always available. The echocardiogram may be negative in right-sided endocarditis, prosthetic valves endocarditis, and sudden-onset, rapidly progressive endocarditis, such as that caused by Gram-negative bacilli.

Treatment

Because of the presence of vegetations consisting of fibrin/platelets/bacteria and persistent bacteraemia, a synergistic combination of antimicrobial agents to achieve bactericidal activity is usually indicated[5, 6]. For example, staphylococcal endocarditis is best treated with high doses of flucloxacillin (i.v., 2 g 4-hourly) and an aminoglycoside, e.g. gentamicin (i.v., 80–120 mg 8-hourly), but if the isolate is methicillin resistant a glycopeptide, i.e. vancomycin (i.v., usually 1 g 12-hourly) or teicoplanin, is substituted for flucloxacillin. Streptococcal endo-carditis is treated with benzylpenicillin (i.v., 1.2 g 4-hourly) or ampicillin (i.v., 2 g 4-hourly) plus gentamicin (i.v., 80 mg 12-hourly), if caused by enterococci and aminoglycoside sensitive[5]. Single daily dosage of gentamicin is not routine in the treatment of endocarditis except where there is poor renal function, and dosing with twice- or thrice-daily regimens leads to accumulation, confirmed following assays of blood levels. The choice of agent and the duration of therapy are dependent on the aetiology, susceptibility of the organism to antibiotics, and the initial response to antibiotics. Apart from selected cases (e.g. endocarditis due to streptococcal strains very sensitive to penicillin, which depending on other factors may be treated for 2 weeks), intravenous followed by oral treatment for 4 weeks or more is the norm[5]. The response to therapy should be monitored clinically and repeat TOE may be useful in monitoring the size of vegetations; a cardiac surgeon should be involved early in management, especially if the response to antibiotics is slow indicating persistent infection, or if there are complications such as a paravalvular abscess. Regular serum assays of amino-glycosides such as gentamicin and vancomycin or, occasionally, teicoplanin should also be carried out to minimize toxicity[5, 6] and to confirm therapeutic blood levels, but serum bactericidal tests or back-titrations are no longer considered necessary[5].

Prophylaxis

The rationale for using antibiotics to prevent infective endocarditis has been succinctly reviewed elsewhere[7]. At-risk patients include those with underlying cardiac conditions (especially prosthetic valves, previous infective endocarditis, cyanotic congenital heart disease, patent ductus arteriosus and aortic or mitral valve stenosis or regurgitation) undergoing dental or surgical procedures. Guide-lines drawn up by relevant experts are available[8] and those for patients undergoing general anaesthesia are included in Table 13.1. It is important to remember, however, that antibacterial agents used for routine surgical prophylaxis (e.g. cefuroxime and metronidazole) to prevent intra-abdominal infection caused by Gram-negative bacilli and anaerobes, as discussed in Chapters 5 and 9, are not optimal for the prevention of infective endocarditis.

It is likely that UK, European and North American guidelines on prophylaxis will undergo further changes as evidence continues to mount suggesting that many patients currently receiving prophylaxis for dental procedures do not need it. It is now being suggested that only patients with a prosthetic value or previous endocarditis undergoing tooth extractions or gingival surgery justify prophylaxis[9]. However, ICU practitioners should continue to follow current guidelines[8, 9] until these are amended by relevant authorities.

Myocardial abscess
Presentation

The presentation of this uncommon condition is often quite subtle, and may be diagnosed only at autopsy, or manifest as part of a disseminated infection with myocardial involvement (e.g. staphylococcal bacteraemia, candidaemia), or be diagnosed following complications such as tamponade, haemopericardium and purulent pericarditis[1].

Diagnosis

Blood cultures are positive in the majority of cases, except with fungal infection. Non-specific electrocardiogram (ECG) changes such as first-degree heart block should prompt further investigation with echocardiography and computed tomography (CT) or magnetic resonance imaging (MRI).

Treatment

Surgical intervention for drainage, or valve replacement, if a paravalvular abscess has developed, together with at least 4 weeks of appropriate parenteral anti-

Table 13.1   Recommendations[a] for the prevention of infective endocarditis in patients requiring general anaesthesia.

Clinical circumstance	Recommended antibiotic(s)
Dental or upper respiratory tract surgery Standard prophylaxis in patients requiring a general anaesthetic, who are not allergic to penicillin and who have not had a penicillin in the last month	Ampicillin/amoxycillin, i.v., 1 g plus gentamicin, i.v., 120 mg, at induction plus amoxycillin, orally, 500 mg 6 hours later
Patients who have had penicillin recently or who are allergic to penicillin	Vancomycin[b], i.v., 1 g, plus gentamicin, i.v., 120 mg at induction
Genitourinary, obstetric/gynaecological and gastrointestinal procedures or surgery Standard prophylaxis in patients who are not allergic to penicillin and who have not had a penicillin in the last month	Ampicillin/amoxycillin, i.v., 1 g, plus gentamicin, i.v., 120 mg, at induction plus amoxycillin, orally, 500 mg 6 hours later
Patients who have had penicillin recently or who are allergic to penicillin	Vancomycin[b], i.v., 1 g, plus gentamicin, i.v., 120 mg at induction

[a] Consult reference 8 and antibiotic data sheets for full details and methods of administration.
[b] Teicoplanin or clindamycin may be substituted for vancomycin.

biotics (e.g. flucloxacillin, i.v., 2 g 6-hourly) are recommended. The outcome will depend upon the size and number of the abscesses, the underlying health of the patient, delay in instituting appropriate antibiotics, aetiology and the development of complications.

Pericarditis

Pericarditis and myocarditis may be non-infective in aetiology (e.g. associated with uraemia or connective tissue disorders) or manifest as part of a generalized infection, with signs and symptoms elsewhere. Viruses are the commonest cause but tuberculosis should also be considered. Purulent pericarditis requiring drainage, although less common, may, however, require management in the ICU.

Presentation

The classical features of fever, chest pain and friction rubs may be absent in patients with purulent pericarditis, particularly after recent antimicrobial therapy, or following cardiac surgery when the pericardium is left open[10]. A high index of suspicion is required in patients following recent surgery, patients who are immunosuppressed, or patients with a history of recent sepsis at another site (e.g. lung).

Diagnosis

The chest X-ray and ECG are usually abnormal but the findings are non-specific and are often recognized only retrospectively. Two-dimensional echo-cardiography will identify the presence of excess pericardial fluid and may be able to distinguish fibropurulent from transudative fluid; TOE is especially useful in the postoperative cardiac surgery patient or in patients with prosthetic valves[10]. A CT or MRI scan is more sensitive in detecting pericarditis in areas inaccessible to echocardiography and pericardiocentesis will confirm the diagnosis, obtain fluid to determine the microbial aetiology and help relieve cardiac tamponade. *Streptococcus pneumoniae*, staphylococci and other streptococci are the commonest causes of bacterial pericarditis but Gram-negative bacilli and meningococci are also implicated[10].

Treatment

Drainage and antibiotics are the key to effective management. Drainage procedures, which may require the expertise of a cardiac surgeon, include pericardiocentesis, pericardiostomy with tube drainage, or the creation of a pericardial window. A pericardiectomy may be required for persistent infection and to avoid constriction. Parenteral antibiotics are required for at least 2 weeks or longer if drainage is not complete, and the choice of antibiotic will depend upon the aetiology, e.g. benzylpenicillin (i.v., 1.8 g 6-hourly) for pneumococcal or meningococcal infection, flucloxacillin (i.v., 2 g 6-hourly) for sensitive staphylococci.

Myocarditis

The true incidence of myocarditis is difficult to determine because of major difficulties in diagnosis. Myocarditis due to infectious agents is the commonest form and may be caused by bacteria, rickettsia and protozoa but enteroviruses are the commonest aetiological agents (Table 13.2). There may be an interval between the initial systemic infection and the development of myocarditis and this is because the pathogenesis is believed to be due to cell-mediated immuno-logical reactions to cell surface changes or to new antigens[11]. Drug hyper-sensitivity reactions (e.g. to amitriptyline, phenytoin, spironolactone) and other causes of inflammation such as radiation also cause myocarditis.

Presentation

The clinical spectrum of illness is variable but fever, dyspnoea (due to heart failure), chest pain (due to associated pericarditis) and palpitations (due to arrhythmias) are the main clinical features.

Table 13.2 Some features of the infectious causes of myocarditis (based on reference 11).

Aetiological agent	Clinical and other features
Viral	
Coxsackie A and B (enteroviruses)	Pleurisy, myalgia, arthralgia and upper respiratory tract symptoms
CMV	Usually only in immunosuppressed patients
Influenza virus	Usually with pre-existing cardiovascular disease
HIV	Progressive dilated cardiomyopathy when CD4 counts are low, but often asymptomatic
Non-viral	
Diphtheria	Heart involved in 20%; toxin inhibits protein synthesis
Group A streptococci	Part of rheumatic fever; may get pancarditis
Leptospirosis	High fatality rate
Lyme disease	Heart block a particular feature
Trypanosomiasis	Occurs in Central and South America with ventricular dilatation and fibrosis

HIV, human immunodeficiency virus; CMV, cytomegalovirus.

Diagnosis

The above symptoms with or without abnormal physical signs on clinical examination together with non-specific findings on ECG (e.g. ST segment and T wave changes), chest X-ray (e.g. cardiomegaly), echocardiography (e.g. impaired systolic contraction) and radionuclide imaging are all suggestive of a myocardial abnormality. Echocardiography is probably the most useful non-invasive investigation[11]. A specific diagnosis is, however, dependent on endomyocardial biopsy with histological examination and virological studies. Routine viral serology to detect a fourfold increase in antibodies may be helpful. Raised IgM titres to Coxsackie B (one of the enteroviral causes) are diagnostic in the early stages but the development of DNA techniques such as *in situ* hybridization of muscle tissue (when a myocardial biopsy is feasible) enables a diagnosis to be made during most stages of the illness and may be useful during follow-up[12]. This technology is not available in all centres and should be discussed with a virologist or microbiologist.

Treatment

Underlying heart failure should be treated with conventional agents, e.g. diuretics, inotropic agents, angiotensin-converting enzyme inhibitors, digoxin and antiarrhythmic agents as required. Ribavirin and interferon have been advocated as antiviral agents for this condition but with conflicting results, and because of the histological similarities between viral myocarditis and heart transplant rejection, immunosuppression with prednisone or azathioprine has also been proposed, but there is little convincing evidence of effectiveness[12]. The 5-year mortality rate is reported to be in the order of 50–60% and this condition is increasingly recognized as a cause of unexpected death in athletes[11].

SURGICAL INFECTIONS

The complexity of many cardiac and vascular surgery procedures, and the presence of chronic underlying diseases such as peripheral vascular disease, mean that infection after cardiac or vascular surgery is associated with significant mortality, organ dysfunction and prolonged hospital stay. As well as daily monitoring of such parameters as cardiac index, immediate postoperative Acute Physiology and Chronic Health Evaluation (APACHE) II scores are predictive of septic complications following cardiac surgery, especially a score of 19 or more on the first postoperative day[13]. In a recent study, 20% of 605 patients undergoing cardiac surgery developed nosocomial infection; 75% of the Gram-negative bacteria responsible were classified as antibiotic resistant, and the mortality rate of patients with infection was 11.5%, significantly greater than that of non-infected patients[14]. Minimizing the duration of surgery by good technique, avoiding the use of unnecessary postoperative antibiotics, decreasing the duration of central venous, urinary or other catheters, and ensuring that preoperative prophylactic antibiotics are administered, all contribute to reducing postoperative infection.

Prosthetic valve endocarditis
The approach to the diagnosis, management and prevention of prosthetic valve endocarditis is similar to that described earlier. The aetiology of early prosthetic valve endocarditis, e.g. less than 3 months after surgery, is dominated by staphylococci, whereas that causing late-onset infection, e.g. 3 months or later after surgery, is similar to native valve endocarditis when streptococci pre-dominate. Surgical intervention to replace an infected prosthetic valve should be considered early before it becomes technically difficult, and the duration of antibiotic treatment is months rather than weeks.

Mediastinitis
This is one of the most feared complications following cardiac surgery. The incidence is approximately 2% but varies with the surgical procedure, the patient population and whether or not the internal mammary artery is used for revascularization, as this vessel is a major blood supply to the sternum[15].

Presentation
Fever (especially if persistent), sternal pain or tenderness, wound inflammation and the presence of pus at the operative site are all suggestive of mediastinitis.

The index of suspicion is especially high in those patients at greatest risk[15, 16], as outlined in Table 13.3.

Diagnosis

The clinical features may suggest the diagnosis. Chest X-ray and thoracic CT may confirm the presence of pus beneath the sternum. Pus or necrotic tissue obtained at exploration for culture is essential as wound swabs may reflect superficial skin or wound flora only. Gram-positive cocci such as *Staphylococcus aureus* are the commonest cause but mixed infections involving Gram-positive and Gram-negative bacteria, e.g. *Acinetobacter* spp. and *Pseudomonas aeruginosa*, are increasingly recognized[15]. Coagulase-negative staphylococci (e.g. *Staphylococcus epidermidis*), which are usually multiply antibiotic resistant and which may be dismissed as contaminants, may also cause mediastinitis[16]. Outbreaks or mini-epidemics of infection caused by uncommon bacteria suggest a common source and suboptimal control of infection procedures; a recent outbreak due to *Rhodococcus bronchialis*, a Gram-positive bacillus, was traced to a contaminated water bath used to carry out clotting times[17]. Finally, repeat blood cultures are essential in confirming a diagnosis, indicating the severity of infection or a distant source, and in guiding the use of appropriate antibiotics.

Treatment

Urgent exploration of the wound with removal of sternal wires and necrotic tissue is essential and helps confirm a microbiological diagnosis by providing deep tissue or pus for culture. Antibiotics, e.g. flucloxacillin (i.v., 2 g 6-hourly) and fusidic acid (orally, 500 mg 6-hourly) for staphylococcal infection, are

Table 13.3   Risk factors for mediastinitis.

Host factors
Obesity
Diabetes
Female sex
Malnutrition

Perioperative factors
Emergency procedures
Intra-aortic balloon pump
Bilateral use of internal mammary arteries for revascularization
Multiple blood transfusion (>10 units)

Postoperative factors
Renal dialysis
External cardiac massage

required for approximately 6 weeks, especially if sternal bony infection is confirmed. Sternectomy and costal cartilage resection with transposition of muscle or omentum may be necessary in the management of chronic infection. The hospital mortality rate is 10–15% and death is often due to multiple organ failure[15].

Infected pacemakers

The use of permanent pacemakers has significantly improved the management of symptomatic bradycardia and heart block, and in general the risk of infectious complications remains low at 1–6%[1]. The development of pacemaker infections will be determined by surgical technique or expertise, certain predisposing factors, e.g. prolonged use of an external pacemaker, and whether manipulation of the pacemaker leads occurs following implantation.

Presentation

Local redness, tenderness, purulent discharge, wound breakdown, skin necrosis or a discharging sinus are amongst the presenting signs and symptoms. Pacemaker dysfunction, if the leads have been manipulated, may also be a feature and systemic illness (e.g. rigors) may indicate the presence of bacteraemia.

Diagnosis

The presenting clinical features together with the results of culture of fluid, pus and blood will confirm a diagnosis; echocardiography should be conducted if endocarditis is suspected. The majority of infections are caused by *S. aureus* but if infection occurs some time after insertion, i.e. over a month, coagulase-negative staphylococci and Gram-negative bacilli may also be isolated. In up to half of cases, however, no organism is identified mainly due to recent empirical antibiotic therapy[18].

Treatment

Localized infection may be adequately treated with parenteral antibiotics alone, e.g. flucloxacillin (i.v., 1 g 6-hourly) if caused by a methicillin-sensitive *S. aureus*. In patients with bacteraemia, accompanying endocarditis or migrated leads, treatment involves surgical removal of the pacemaker and leads, with complete debridement of all inflammatory tissue and foreign material from the pacemaker pocket, with antibiotics[18]. Where bacteraemia or endocarditis has been diagnosed or suspected, antibiotics should be continued for 6 weeks, but otherwise 2 weeks of antibiotic treatment is probably sufficient.

Aortic and other vascular graft infections

The management of the infected vascular graft poses considerable challenges to the many different specialties. The incidence of infection is low (about 2%), but these infections are associated with high mortality, significant morbidity and considerable expense due to the many investigations undertaken, the requirement for repeated surgical interventions and prolonged antibiotic treatment. A number of factors[19] influencing the likelihood of prosthetic grafts becoming infected have been identified:

1. Failure to use antibiotic prophylaxis during the initial surgical procedure
2. Poor immune status or chronic illnesses in the patient
3. Prosthetic lower limb extremity grafts compared with abdominal grafts
4. Extra-anatomical bypass grafts
5. Infected groin wounds

Low-grade pathogens such as coagulase-negative staphylococci (e.g. *S. epidermidis*) may be found in the walls of diseased arteries or regional lymph nodes and may subsequently colonize and infect the prosthesis. These organisms adhere well to graft materials due to the production of extracellular polysaccharides, which adversely affect local immune function such as the migration of inflammatory cells. These factors together with multiple antibiotic resistance usually render treatment with antibiotics alone unsuccessful.

Presentation
The interval between the original procedure and the emergence of infection may range from weeks to 10 years or more. Clinical signs and symptoms will vary depending on the location of the graft, the extent of infection and whether complications such as thrombosis have occurred. Fever, groin infection, a false aneurysm, thrombosis of one limb, septic emboli and gastrointestinal haemorrhage (if an aortoenteric fistula is present) are features of infected vascular grafts[20]. An infected vascular graft should always be considered in any patient with a fever and a history of previous vascular surgery.

Diagnosis
An extensive investigation may be precluded by the necessity for emergency surgery in those patients presenting with major haemorrhage or ischaemia. Clinical features together with a range of possible investigations such as ultrasonography, angiography, CT and nuclear scans (e.g. gallium) will often confirm the presence and extent of infection[20]. A microbiological diagnosis is often not possible until material is obtained at surgery, and the results of culture of superficial swabs or even fluid draining from a sinus tract may be misleading. Furthermore, patients may have received antibiotics from general practitioners or a referring doctor before the diagnosis is confirmed and this partly explains the high incidence of negative cultures.

Treatment
The complexities and options for surgical management are beyond the scope of this text. The anatomical location of infection and the availability of homologous graft material largely determine the surgical strategy and outcome in the management of aortic infections[21]. The best results are usually obtained following the complete removal of the infected graft. Peripheral graft infections

may occasionally be managed conservatively if there is no involvement of the anastomosis, if a pseudoaneurysm is not present and if the artery containing the vascular graft remains patent. Some patients (e.g. the debilitated elderly) may not be fit for further surgery and this will also influence approaches to management. Removal of the infected graft reduces the burden of infected necrotic tissue, facilitates the insertion of new graft and provides material for culture, which is crucial, as antibiotics chosen according to sensitivity results need to be continued for months.

Empirical therapy should usually include a glycopeptide, e.g. vancomycin (i.v., 1 g 12-hourly) or teicoplanin (i.v., 200–400 mg daily) to cover Gram-positive bacteria; metronidazole (i.v., 500 mg 8-hourly) to cover anaerobic bacteria and a third-generation cephalosporin, preferably with antipseudomonal activity such as ceftazidime (i.v., 2 g 8-hourly), or a fluoroquinolone such as ciprofloxacin (i.v., 400 mg 12-hourly) to cover aerobic Gram-negative bacilli. Definitive antibiotic therapy should be discussed with a medical microbiologist or infectious disease physician following the results of culture and antibiotic sensitivity testing as treatment needs to be continued for prolonged periods and antibiotic assays of aminoglycosides or glycopeptides must be carried out at regular intervals.

Key points

- Infections of the cardiovascular system are important because of the complexity of their management and the need to involve many disciplines.
- Infective endocarditis should be suspected in any patient with fever and a murmur.
- Myocarditis and pericarditis caused by enteroviruses are usually self-limiting.
- Mediastinitis caused by unusual bacteria may indicate a common source of infection in the operating theatre or ICU environment.
- Antibiotics alone are usually inadequate in the management of infected aortic or peripheral vascular grafts.

REFERENCES

1. Kearney RA, Eisen HJ, Wolf JE (1994) Non-valvular infections of the cardiovascular system. *Annals of Internal Medicine* **121**: 219–230.
2. La Scol A, Raoult D (1999) Culture of *Bartonella quintana* and *Bartonella henselae* from human samples: a 5-year experience (1993 to 1998). *Journal of Clinical Microbiology* **31**: 1899–1905.
3. Hoen B, Béguinot I, Rabaud C *et al.* (1996) The Duke criteria for diagnosing infective endocarditis are specific: analysis of 100 patients with acute fever of unknown origin. *Clinical Infectious Diseases* **23**: 298–302.

4. Olaison L, Hogevik H (1996) Comparison of the von Reyn and Duke criteria for the diagnosis of infective endocarditis: a critical analysis of 161 episodes. *Scandinavian Journal of Infectious Diseases* **28**: 399–406.

5. Working Party of the British Society for Antimicrobial Chemotherapy (1998) Antibiotic treatment of streptococcal, enterococcal and staphylococcal endocarditis. *Heart* **79**: 207–210.

6. Littler WA (1998) Antimicrobial therapy for bacterial endocarditis on native valves. *Journal of Infection* **36**: 137–139.

7. Durack DT (1995) Prevention of infective endocarditis. *New England Journal of Medicine* **332**: 38–44.

8. British Society of Antimicrobial Chemotherapy Working Party (1993) Recommendations for endocarditis prophylaxis. *Journal of Antimicrobial Chemotherapy* **31**: 437–438.

9. Durack DT (1998) Antibiotics for prevention of endocarditis during dentistry: time to scale back. *Annals of Internal Medicine* **129**: 829–831.

10. Park S, Bayer AS (1992) Purulent pericarditis. In: *Current Clinical Topics in Infectious Diseases*, vol. 12 (eds Remington JS, Swartz MN), pp 56–82. Blackwell Scientific Publications, Cambridge, MA.

11. Brodison A, Swann JW (1998) Myocarditis: a review. *Journal of Infection* **37**: 99–103.

12. Richardson P, Why H (1997) Clinical spectrum of viral heart disease. In: *Viral Infections of the Heart* (ed. Banatvalva JE), pp 59–81. Edward Arnold, London.

13. Kreuzer E, Kääb S, Pilz G et al. (1992) Early prediction of septic complications after cardiac surgery by APACHE II score. *European Journal of Cardiothoracic Surgery* **6**: 524–529.

14. Kollef MH, Sharpless L, Vlasnik J et al. (1997) The impact of nosocomial infections on patient outcomes following cardiac surgery. *Chest* **112**: 666–675.

15. Ulicny KS, Hiratzka LF (1991) The risk factors of median sternotomy infection; a current review. *Journal of Cardiac Surgery* **6**: 338–351.

16. Ståhle E, Tammelin A, Bergström R et al. (1997) Sternal wound complications – incidence, microbiology and risk factors. *European Journal of Cardiothoracic Surgery* **11**: 1146–1153.

17. Richet HM, Craven PC, Brown JM et al. (1991) A cluster of *Rhodococcus (Gordona) bronchialis* sternal-wound infections after coronary-artery bypass surgery. *New England Journal of Medicine* **324**: 104–109.

18. Vogt PR, Sagdic K, Lachat M et al. (1996) Surgical management of infected permanent transvenous pacemaker systems. *Journal of Cardiac Surgery* **11**: 180–186.

19. Bandyk DF (1991) Vascular graft infections; epidemiology, microbiology, pathogenesis, and prevention. In: *Complications in Vascular Surgery* (eds Bernhard VM, Towne JB), pp 223–224. Quality Medical Publishing, St Louis, MO.

20. Faggioli GL, Ricotta JJ (1992) Aortic graft infections. In: *Current Critical Problems in Vascular Surgery*, vol. 4 (ed. Veith FJ), pp 371–380. Quality Medical Publishing, St Louis, MO.

21. von Segesser LK, Vogt P, Genoni M et al. (1997) The infected aorta. *Journal of Cardiac Surgery* **12**: 256–261.

Index

Note: Page references in *italics* refer to Figures; those in **bold** refer to Tables

219

Commissioning Editor: Serena Bureau
Project Development Manager: Kim Benson
Project Manager: Cheryl Brant
Production Manager: Mark Sanderson
Designer: Ian Spick

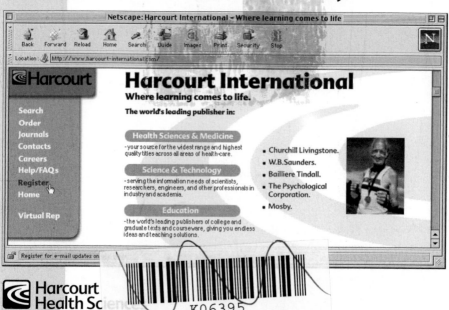